Praise for Liz Neporent's Other Books

Fitness For Dummies with Suzanne Schlosberg:

"This book will come in handy for those of us who don't know a fat gram from Phil Gramm or a donut from a bagel. Now all I need to know is how to look cool and studly in the gym while sweating profusely."

> — Steve Elling, *Raleigh News & Observer*

"This book is a joy to read — written with wit and style, it comes as a welcome reassurance that both razor sharp accuracy and first-rate writing can co-exist in the same package."

> — Jonathan Bowden, M.A.C.S.C.S., Senior Faculty, Equinox Fitness Training Institute and Contributing Editor, *Fitness* magazine

"*Fitness For Dummies* is a smart buy for the exercise enthusiast. It's the fitness equivalent of carbo-loading."

> — *Orange County Register*

"This is one of the most comprehensive, authoritative — and entertaining — fitness books I've ever seen."

> — *Men's Fitness* magazine

"The exercise content and evaluations in this book are outstanding. Liz and Suzanne are the ultimate professionals, and *Fitness For Dummies* will help all exercisers maximize their potential."

> — *Fitness* magazine

"*Fitness For Dummies* is the definitive book for people who would like to achieve a stronger, healthier body."

> — Mark Allen, Six-Time Ironman Champion

"Suzanne and Liz have created an insider's guide through the maze of misinformation about fitness. Before you buy an exercise gadget, a gym membership, or a fitness video, read this book!"

> — *Women's Sports & Fitness* magazine

"*Fitness For Dummies* is a real rarity: a fitness book written by fitness writers — two of the best. It's full of smart, jargon-free, common-sense advice for anyone who's interested in fitness. These two are not afraid to tell the truth. It's like getting the word from a trusted friend."

— *Shape* magazine

"From dispelling myths such as how we really burn fat to a comprehensive look at every choice of equipment on the market today, this book becomes a trustworthy, truly helpful guide to getting in shape."

— Diana Nyad, World Record Holder, Longest Swim in History

Weight Training For Dummies with Suzanne Schlosberg:

"From etiquette to execution, all of weight training do's and don'ts are here, presented just as we dummies like it — straightforward and with loads of humor. Going to the gym has never been this much fun."

— Alex Harvey, Lifestyle/Entertainment Editor, *The Birmingham News*

"Once again you can benefit from the knowledge of two fitness insiders. *Weight Training For Dummies* provides a fun, easy-to-follow guide on the best way to fast results: strength training. Armed with info on gym jargon, etiquette, myth busting, choosing a trainer and more, you'll never be intimidated by a weight room again."

— Peg Moline, Editorial Director, *Shape* magazine

"I highly recommend this exercise bible: it's for anyone who's never walked into a weight room, but more importantly, it's for anyone who's ever walked out of a weight room feeling frustrated, injured, overlooked, or self-conscious. *Weight Training For Dummies* is an information-packed, educational, accessible accomplishment."

— Nicole Dorsey, M.S., Fitness Director, *Fitness* magazine

"Written by humans for humans, this clearly written and comprehensive book (of course grunting is covered) shows how anyone can make weight training a safe and beneficial part of their fitness life. *Weight Training For Dummies* is definitely a smart choice."

— Peter Sikowitz, Editor-in-Chief, *Men's Fitness* magazine

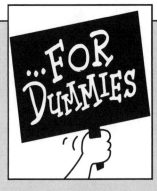
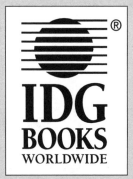

Fitness Walking

FOR

DUMMIES®

Fitness Walking FOR DUMMIES®

by Liz Neporent

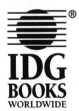

IDG Books Worldwide, Inc.
An International Data Group Company

Foster City, CA ◆ Chicago, IL ◆ Indianapolis, IN ◆ New York, NY

Fitness Walking For Dummies®

Published by
IDG Books Worldwide, Inc.
An International Data Group Company
919 E. Hillsdale Blvd.
Suite 400
Foster City, CA 94404
www.idgbooks.com (IDG Books Worldwide Web site)
www.dummies.com (Dummies Press Web site)

Library of Congress Catalog Card No.: 99-66421

ISBN: 0-7645-5192-2

Printed in the United States of America

10 9 8 7 6 5 4 3 2 1

1B/QS/RS/ZZ/IN

Distributed in the United States by IDG Books Worldwide, Inc.

Distributed by CDG Books Canada Inc. for Canada; by Transworld Publishers Limited in the United Kingdom; by IDG Norge Books for Norway; by IDG Sweden Books for Sweden; by IDG Books Australia Publishing Corporation Pty. Ltd. for Australia and New Zealand; by TransQuest Publishers Pte Ltd. for Singapore, Malaysia, Thailand, Indonesia, and Hong Kong; by Gotop Information Inc. for Taiwan; by ICG Muse, Inc. for Japan; by Intersoft for South Africa; by Eyrolles for France; by International Thomson Publishing for Germany, Austria and Switzerland; by Distribuidora Cuspide for Argentina; by LR International for Brazil; by Galileo Libros for Chile; by Ediciones ZETA S.C.R. Ltda. for Peru; by WS Computer Publishing Corporation, Inc., for the Philippines; by Contemporanea de Ediciones for Venezuela; by Express Computer Distributors for the Caribbean and West Indies; by Micronesia Media Distributor, Inc. for Micronesia; by Chips Computadoras S.A. de C.V. for Mexico; by Editorial Norma de Panama S.A. for Panama; by American Bookshops for Finland.

For general information on IDG Books Worldwide's books in the U.S., please call our Consumer Customer Service department at 800-762-2974. For reseller information, including discounts and premium sales, please call our Reseller Customer Service department at 800-434-3422.

For information on where to purchase IDG Books Worldwide's books outside the U.S., please contact our International Sales department at 317-596-5530 or fax 317-596-5692.

For consumer information on foreign language translations, please contact our Customer Service department at 1-800-434-3422, fax 317-596-5692, or e-mail rights@idgbooks.com.

For information on licensing foreign or domestic rights, please phone +1-650-655-3109.

For sales inquiries and special prices for bulk quantities, please contact our Sales department at 650-655-3200 or write to the address above.

For information on using IDG Books Worldwide's books in the classroom or for ordering examination copies, please contact our Educational Sales department at 800-434-2086 or fax 317-596-5499.

For press review copies, author interviews, or other publicity information, please contact our Public Relations department at 650-655-3000 or fax 650-655-3299.

For authorization to photocopy items for corporate, personal, or educational use, please contact Copyright Clearance Center, 222 Rosewood Drive, Danvers, MA 01923, or fax 978-750-4470.

About the Author

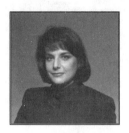

Liz Neporent is a certified trainer and president of Plus One Health Management, a fitness consulting company in New York City. Her job is to make sure that fitness center members at more than a dozen centers in hotels and corporations throughout New York are happy, motivated, and exercising on a regular basis.

Liz holds a master's degree in exercise physiology and is certified by the American Council on Exercise, the American College of Sports Medicine, the National Strength and Conditioning Association, and the National Academy of Sports Medicine. She is coauthor of the *Buns of Steel: Total Body Workout* and *Abs of Steel* videos and *Weight Training For Dummies*. She is also the coauthor of *Fitness For Dummies*. Additionally, she is the gear editor for *Shape* and a regular contributor to *The New York Times*. She appears regularly on TV and radio as an authority on fitness and exercise.

Liz is an avid runner, hiker, and walker. She has competed in more than two dozen marathons and ultra-marathons and once power walked over 40 miles. She is also devoted to sports climbing, Pilates, and weight training. She lives in New York City, where she walks to work and takes daily walks with her husband, Jay Shafran, and her greyhound, Zoomer.

ABOUT IDG BOOKS WORLDWIDE

Welcome to the world of IDG Books Worldwide.

IDG Books Worldwide, Inc., is a subsidiary of International Data Group, the world's largest publisher of computer-related information and the leading global provider of information services on information technology. IDG was founded more than 30 years ago by Patrick J. McGovern and now employs more than 9,000 people worldwide. IDG publishes more than 290 computer publications in over 75 countries. More than 90 million people read one or more IDG publications each month.

Launched in 1990, IDG Books Worldwide is today the #1 publisher of best-selling computer books in the United States. We are proud to have received eight awards from the Computer Press Association in recognition of editorial excellence and three from Computer Currents' First Annual Readers' Choice Awards. Our best-selling *...For Dummies®* series has more than 50 million copies in print with translations in 31 languages. IDG Books Worldwide, through a joint venture with IDG's Hi-Tech Beijing, became the first U.S. publisher to publish a computer book in the People's Republic of China. In record time, IDG Books Worldwide has become the first choice for millions of readers around the world who want to learn how to better manage their businesses.

Our mission is simple: Every one of our books is designed to bring extra value and skill-building instructions to the reader. Our books are written by experts who understand and care about our readers. The knowledge base of our editorial staff comes from years of experience in publishing, education, and journalism — experience we use to produce books to carry us into the new millennium. In short, we care about books, so we attract the best people. We devote special attention to details such as audience, interior design, use of icons, and illustrations. And because we use an efficient process of authoring, editing, and desktop publishing our books electronically, we can spend more time ensuring superior content and less time on the technicalities of making books.

You can count on our commitment to deliver high-quality books at competitive prices on topics you want to read about. At IDG Books Worldwide, we continue in the IDG tradition of delivering quality for more than 30 years. You'll find no better book on a subject than one from IDG Books Worldwide.

John Kilcullen
Chairman and CEO
IDG Books Worldwide, Inc.

Steven Berkowitz
President and Publisher
IDG Books Worldwide, Inc.

WINNER

Eighth Annual Computer Press Awards ≥1992

WINNER

Ninth Annual Computer Press Awards ≥1993

WINNER

Tenth Annual Computer Press Awards ≥1994

WINNER

Eleventh Annual Computer Press Awards ≥1995

Dedication

This book is dedicated to my husband, Jay Shafran, and in loving memory of Donna Marie McGovern.

Author's Acknowledgments

Many thanks to my Plus One partners, Jay Shafran, Mike Motta, and Bill Horne. Thanks also to the entire Plus One staff with special thanks to Grace De Simone, Holly Byrne, Baze Amiri, Lemont Platt, Bob Welter, Jamie Macdonald, and Tom Maraday. And, as always, thanks to the individual site managers for making my job so easy and giving me the time to do all of my extracurricular projects: John Buzzerio, Shel Bibbey, Kathleen Troy, Jason Ferrara, Terry Certain, Nancy Ngai, Nancy Belli, Mary Franz, Laura Girodano, Tom McCann, and Carrie Wujick.

I am indebted to Mitchel Gray, my photographer, and all the models depicted throughout this book: Nancy Ngai, Shel Bibbey, Terry Certain, Aja Certain, Annemarie Scarammucia, Melody Fadness, Yvonne Mitchell, Chris Stothard, Stacy Collins, Val Towne, James Jankiewicz, Jay Shafran, Doris Shafran, Melissa Saxon, Patty Buttenheim, Sunshine Hopkins, and Jane Scott.

To my parents, sister, brothers, nieces, nephews, and all my in-laws — thanks for your encouragement. Ditto to my good friends Patty Buttenheim, Gina Allchin, Norman Zinker, Mary Duffy, and Suzanne Schlosberg. Thanks to Frank Tirelli, Lucy McGovern, Pam DiPietro, and David Wildstein for helping out with organization and proofreading.

Thanks also to Jennifer Kries, my Method instructor and good friend, and my climbing gurus and best buds, Stephen Harris and Ivan Greene. My undying gratitude to Eli Jacobson for teaching me everything he knows about tax law and exercise.

A very special thanks to my husband, Jay Shafran, who is without a doubt the most supportive person on the face of the earth. (Can you please take the dog for a walk while I finish this up?)

Publisher's Acknowledgments

We're proud of this book; please register your comments through our IDG Books Worldwide Online Registration Form located at `http://my2cents.dummies.com`.

Some of the people who helped bring this book to market include the following:

Acquisitions, Editorial, and Media Development

Editors: Andrea Boucher, Tina Sims

Acquisitions Editor: Stacy S. Collins

General Reviewers: Gina Allchin, Marlisa Brown, Holly Byrne, Grace DeSimone, Risa Halpern, Richard Miller, Lemont Platt, Sarah Bowen Shea

Acquisitions Coordinators: Lisa Roule, Jonathan Malysiak

Editorial Managers: Jennifer Ehrlich, Pam Mourouzis

Editorial Assistants: Laura Jefferson, Carol Strickland

Production

Project Coordinator: Regina Snyder

Layout and Graphics: Amy Adrian, Clint Lahnen, Shelley Norris, Barry Offringa, Tracy Oliver, Jill Piscitelli, Brent Savage, Janet Seib, Jacque Schneider, Brian Torwelle, Maggie Ubertini, Dan Whetstine, Erin Zeltner

Photography: Sunstreak Productions, Inc.

Proofreaders: Laura Albert, John Greenough, Arielle Carole Meunelle, Charles Spencer

Indexer: Sherry Massey

Special Help

Kathleen Dobie, Donna Fredericks, Elizabeth Kuball, Patricia Yuu Pan, Janet M. Withers

---

General and Administrative

IDG Books Worldwide, Inc.: John Kilcullen, CEO; Steven Berkowitz, President and Publisher

IDG Books Technology Publishing Group: Richard Swadley, Senior Vice President and Publisher; Walter Bruce III, Vice President and Associate Publisher; Joseph Wikert, Associate Publisher; Mary Bednarek, Branded Product Development Director; Mary Corder, Editorial Director; Barry Pruett, Publishing Manager; Michelle Baxter, Publishing Manager

IDG Books Consumer Publishing Group: Roland Elgey, Senior Vice President and Publisher; Kathleen A. Welton, Vice President and Publisher; Kevin Thornton, Acquisitions Manager; Kristin A. Cocks, Editorial Director

IDG Books Internet Publishing Group: Brenda McLaughlin, Senior Vice President and Publisher; Diane Graves Steele, Vice President and Associate Publisher; Sofia Marchant, Online Marketing Manager

IDG Books Production for Dummies Press: Debbie Stailey, Associate Director of Production; Cindy L. Phipps, Manager of Project Coordination, Production Proofreading, and Indexing; Tony Augsburger, Manager of Prepress, Reprints, and Systems; Laura Carpenter, Production Control Manager; Shelley Lea, Supervisor of Graphics and Design; Debbie J. Gates, Production Systems Specialist; Robert Springer, Supervisor of Proofreading; Kathie Schutte, Production Supervisor

Dummies Packaging and Book Design: Patty Page, Manager, Promotions Marketing

◆

The publisher would like to give special thanks to Patrick J. McGovern, without whom this book would not have been possible.

◆

Contents at a Glance

Cartoons at a Glance

By Rich Tennant

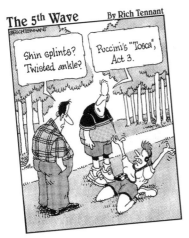

page 147

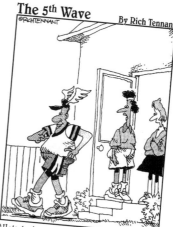

"He's lost 12 lbs. and 3 inches from his waist. Now, if I can just get him to lose that hat."

page 259

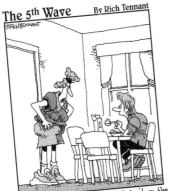

"I know I walk regularly and I do it on the street, but if anyone asks, I'm a fitness-walker, or a power-walker, NOT a street-walker."

page 5

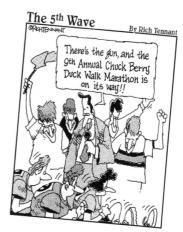

page 91

Fax: 978-546-7747
E-mail: richtennant@the5thwave.com
World Wide Web: www.the5thwave.com

Table of Contents

Introduction

• •

*A*ngel, a woman who attends a weekly Internet chat that I host, used to be very skeptical about using walking to get in shape. I encouraged her for weeks to give it a try, but she didn't believe that something as simple as walking would help her improve her fitness level and lose weight. Finally, thanks to a lot of nagging on my part, she agreed to give it a try. After about eight weeks of steadily and faithfully walking five times a week, she excitedly reported to the group that she had lost 20 pounds. "I can't believe it works, but it definitely does!" she told the group. Now everyone is on board. Each week we all pledge to complete a weekly exercise and diet assignment, which invariably includes an element of walking.

Like Angel, many people have trouble believing that the act of putting one foot in front of the other can be an effective way of exercising. And, just like Angel, those who take those first steps and keep on going almost always come to appreciate the impressive benefits of a walking program. Here are only a few ways that walking can help you:

✔ **Walking is safe and easy to do for nearly everyone, including older folks, pregnant women, and those who are very out of shape.** Almost everyone can start out — and continue — a fitness program with walking. Walking is one of the easiest workouts in the world to continue throughout your entire life.

✔ **You can lose weight by walking.** A large study sponsored by the National Weight Control Registry found that more than 80 percent of long-term "losers" used walking as their primary form of exercise. The faster you walk and the more you weigh, the more calories you will burn. In fact, walking burns about the same number of calories per mile as running.

✔ **Walking is one of the most adaptable workout activities around.** You don't need to walk for an hour straight to make your walking program effective and to achieve your goals. You can accumulate this hour over the course of a day, which means that you can adapt your walking program to fit your lifestyle and schedule. And, because there are four levels of walking, your program can grow with you as your fitness level improves.

✔ **Walking can help you live a longer, healthier life.** The health benefits of walking include decreased blood pressure and an increase in HDL, or "good," cholesterol by up to 6 percent, according to one study performed at the Cooper Institute for Aerobic Research. Scores of studies support the theory that walking just a few miles a week may help prevent heart disease, diabetes, and some forms of cancer.

✔ **Walking is an effective way to preserve bone density and prevent osteoporosis, a disease in which bones become brittle, increasing the likelihood of fractures.** Because walking is a weight-bearing activity, it places stress on your bones and stimulates the growth of bone cells. But because it is low impact — less than half the impact of running — you have little chance of injuring yourself.

✔ **Walking offers emotional benefits.** Study after study has found that it helps counter depression and relieve stress. Walking refreshes the spirit, often giving you a break from your hectic life. It's a wonderful way to stop and smell the roses without actually having to stop!

This is just a snapshot of the things walking can do for you. It seems that nearly every day some new study, some new piece of evidence, is published extolling yet another of walking's virtues.

Perhaps that's why you bought this book. Like 67 million other people in this country who log over 201 million miles a year, you want to take advantage of all of the great things a regular walking program can do for you. Whether you want to improve your health or your appearance, lose weight, get stronger, feel good about yourself, or all of the above, walking can help you get to where you want to go. This book can help you do that by telling you every-thing you need to know about starting and maintaining a walking program.

How to Use This Book

You can use this book in one of two ways:

✔ You can read it from cover to cover to discover everything you need to know about starting and maintaining a walking program.

✔ You can use it as a reference to look up specific topics about walking and exercise in general. Novices can look up anything related to walking to help them advance their programs. Experts can use this as a refer-ence to find out about the latest walking-related information.

How This Book is Organized

Fitness Walking For Dummies is divided into four parts. The chapters within each part are grouped together to cover a lot about a general walking-related topic. Read in its entirety, each section gives you a complete overview of this topic. However, you can read each chapter separately to find out about a spe-cific concept. I refer you to other chapters if I cover something in greater detail elsewhere in the book. Here's a brief overview of the four sections:

Part I: Getting Started

In this part, I give you all the information you need to start a walking program. I explain why it's important to know your starting point and to have clear, specific goals for your walking program. I tell you everything you need to know about walking gear, especially walking shoes. I give you the skinny on basic nutrition and then tell you how to eat for optimal walking performance. I explain how to design a walking workout to meet your goals, how to walk safely and stay injury free, and how to deal with walking in all kinds of weather.

Part II: Basic Training

This part starts out with a brief overview of how to structure your warm-up and cool-down. The rest of this part is devoted to the four different levels of walking. Level 1, lifestyle walking, is perfect for exercisers just beginning a walking program. Level 2, fitness walking, picks up the pace for added health benefits and increased weight loss and is the type of walking most exercisers choose as their main form of activity. High-energy walking, Level 3, is similar to race walking, only you don't have to be competitive to reap its calorie-burning, heart-pumping, body-shaping benefits. Finally, for those who like to exercise in the fast lane, Level 4, walk-run, lets you experiment with faster paced walking and running for the ultimate calorie burn without undue risk of injury.

Part III: Beyond the Basics

In this part, I home in on topics that can help your walking program become more interesting and effective. For example, I give you the ten best weight training exercises and the ten best stretches for walkers. You find out how to spice up your routine with advanced techniques, what to do to avoid walking injuries, and what type of program works best for special circumstances like pregnancy and loss of balance as you get older. I also take you step by step through buying and using a treadmill. Finally, I discuss some fun ways to vary your routine by walking on the beach, through the woods, around the mall, or in the swimming pool.

Part IV: Part of Tens

This part is devoted to topics that can help you improve your walking program and, in some cases, your health. I give you ideas for gadgets and gear to enhance your walking experience. I tell you where to find even more information about walking. In conclusion, I provide ten great pieces of advice on how to stay motivated about walking for years to come.

Icons Used in This Book

Throughout this book, I offset some information with a series of icons. When you see an icon, you will know what type of information is coming and that it's so important I'm giving you a heads up. Here's a list of all the icons I use.

This icon lets you know that you're about to encounter some advanced walking terminology, such as "target training zone" or "lactic acid." This information may help you structure your walking program and interpret walking information that you may read elsewhere.

This icon highlights my recommendations on best buys, great products, excellent Web sites, and other walking-related items and issues. Flip to the appendix to find a reference section listing further information on anything that's earned the Dummies Approved label.

The Beware icon warns you about everything from wasting your money to staying safe in certain situations. When you see this icon, pay extra attention to what I'm telling you.

This icon lets you know when I'm about to dispel a common myth about walking or some other topic. For instance, when I dispel the myth throughout this book that running burns more calories than walking, the Myth Buster icon will be there to reinforce the fact that, mile for mile, you burn about the same number of calories walking as you do running.

Whenever I have a good story or real-life example to help illustrate a point, I use the Anecdote icon. My stories range from wacky to inspirational.

This icon highlights good ideas and strategies to help make your walking program more effective. It also flags ideas on how to save money and time.

You see this icon in Chapters 11 and 12. This icon underscores the importance of using good form and technique to increase the effectiveness of your program and to prevent injury.

This icon appears in only Chapters 11 and 12. It suggests that you skip or modify an exercise to accommodate any injuries or joint problems you have, such as a bad back or a sore knee. Even if you don't have any problems, this icon gives you a heads up to take special care during an exercise to protect certain body parts.

Part I
Getting Started

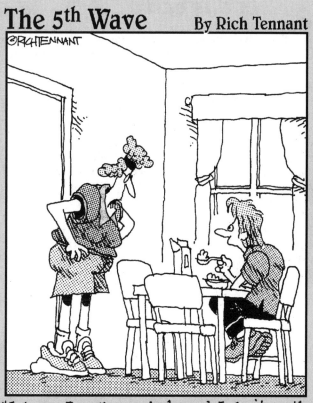

The 5th Wave   By Rich Tennant

"I know I walk regularly and I do it on the street, but if anyone asks, I'm a fitness-walker, or a power-walker, NOT a street-walker."

In this part . . .

1 tell you everything you need to know to personalize and perfect your walking program in this part. Chapter 1 explains the importance of testing your fitness level before you start your walking program and then retesting it periodically. I also give you step-by-step instructions on how to do the tests I recommend. Chapter 2 discusses one of the most important ways to stay pumped about your walking program: goal setting. In Chapter 3, I tell you everything you need to know about walking gear, especially how to buy walking shoes and how to lace them properly. Then, in Chapter 4, I give you a basic nutrition lesson and offer some tips on how to apply these basics to your lifestyle and level of activity. The final chapter in this section focuses on walking logistics. I introduce the different levels of walking, explain how to structure your walking program by using the FIT formula, and give you some tips on how to deal with inclement weather.

Chapter 1

Knowing Your Numbers

. . . .

In This Chapter

▶ Understanding why you need to know your starting point

▶ Determining your risk of cardiovascular disease

▶ Knowing what your resting heart rate and blood pressure mean about your health

▶ Measuring body fat and body mass index (BMI)

▶ Testing your heart, lungs, and endurance

▶ Assessing strength and flexibility

▶ Understanding why you have to retest

▶ Figuring out your personal testing scorecard

. . . .

*W*hen you go out for a walk, certain signposts mark the progress of your workout. For instance, when you walk past the yellow house on the corner of Fair and Franklin, you know that you're about a half mile into your walk. You may also measure your workout progress by how long you've been walking or by how tired you feel at certain points along your route.

To measure the progress of your *entire* fitness program, you can determine some physical and health signposts. That's why you evaluate your fitness level before you begin your walking program. By knowing where you're starting from, you can eventually see how far you've come.

This chapter contains some simple fitness tests you can do yourself. These tests are not pass or fail. Their purpose is to enlighten you about which aspects of your fitness level could stand some improvement.

The tests I've selected are specifically geared toward walkers, but certainly dozens of other evaluations are valid and can give you a reasonably accurate snapshot of your health and physical fitness level. If you find a test somewhere else that you like better than the ones I provide in this chapter, feel free to take it. Record your initial results in the personal testing scorecard (Table 1-1) at the end of this chapter. Use them as a basis of comparison and measure of progress when you compare them to your retest results a few months down the road.

You may want to photocopy the personal testing scorecard (Table 1-1) for family members and friends.

If you do not feel comfortable testing yourself, you can hire a medical and fitness professional to help you with the process. A qualified personal trainer may charge you between $50 and $250 to do a complete fitness evaluation that includes an explanation of the results and some recommendations on how to proceed with your walking and overall workout program.

The tests in this chapter are *not* designed to take the place of a thorough checkup by your doctor. No self-evaluation can ever do that.

To complete these tests, you need about 45 minutes. You also need access to a running track or a measured 1-mile route and the following materials:

- A pen or pencil
- A stopwatch or a watch with a second hand or timer
- A measuring tape
- A calculator
- An exercise mat, thick bath towel, or padded carpet

Understanding Your Risk for Heart Disease

Assessing your risk of developing cardiovascular disease is important to ensure that it's safe for you to begin exercising. By asking yourself a few simple questions and answering them as honestly as possible, you can get a reasonably accurate picture of your cardiac health risk factors.

Answer yes or no to the following questions. Jot your answers down in the margin or on a separate sheet of paper.

- Has a doctor told you that you have some form of heart disease?
- Do you *sometimes* have pains in your heart and chest?
- Do you *sometimes* feel faint or have dizzy spells?
- Has your doctor ever told you that you have high blood pressure?
- Have you gone more than a year without doing regular, vigorous exercise?
- Are you above your optimal weight? (See the section "Figuring Out Your Body Weight and Body Composition," later in this chapter.)

✔ Do you smoke cigarettes or have you smoked in the last two years?

✔ Has your doctor ever told you that you have high cholesterol?

✔ Are you currently taking any prescribed medications?

✔ Were either of your parents or any of your siblings ever diagnosed with heart disease before the age of 60?

✔ Has your doctor ever told you that you have high blood sugar or diabetes?

✔ Do you have severe arthritis or a similar limitation that may prevent you from exercising safely?

✔ Do you have any other condition, problem, or limitation such as chronic back pain or knee pain that may make it unsafe for you to begin an exercise program?

Answering the preceding questions is more than just a way to increase your health awareness. Take a look at the following to determine whether you should consult with your physician before proceeding with an exercise program.

✔ If you answer yes to one or more of the questions and you are over 35 years of age, I recommend seeing a physician for a checkup before you begin exercising.

✔ If you are younger than 35 and answer yes to two or more of the questions, you should also visit your doctor before you begin exercising.

✔ If you are younger than 35 and answered yes to no more than one of the questions, it is probably safe to begin an exercise program.

✔ If you are 45 years or older and haven't had a medical checkup in more than a year, you may want to go ahead and make an appointment with your doctor just to play it safe, even if you didn't answer yes to any of the questions.

The questions in this section are by no means a substitute for medical advice! Many other factors, such as your stress level or the fact that you smoke cigars, may also affect your health and ability to exercise. If you have any reason to think that you may have a condition that can limit your ability to exercise, play it safe and check in with your doctor.

I know that taking this extra step can be a pain because it delays the start of your exercise program, but it ensures that you can exercise safely and comfortably. Besides, most physicians want you to exercise. Even if your doctor finds a problem, she can usually correct it with medication or some other means and get you out and walking in no time.

Determining Your Resting Heart Rate

The average, healthy person has a resting heart rate between 60 and 90 beats per minute (bpm). It may be slower if you're in good physical condition or genetically predisposed to a low heart rate; it may be higher if you're stressed out or you recently had caffeine or smoked a cigarette. Because exercise makes your heart more efficient, your resting heart rate will probably slow down within a few months of beginning your exercise program. It's not uncommon to see drops of 5 to 30 beats per minute as a result of regular exercise.

Here's how to determine your heart rate: Place your watch so that you can look at it easily. Gently press the tips of your middle and index fingers of your right hand against the base of your left wrist directly below your thumb. You should feel a light pulsing sensation; this is your heart rate, also known as your pulse. Count how many beats you feel in one minute and record this number in Table 1-1.

You may also want to check your blood pressure, although this is difficult to do on your own. The average person has a blood pressure close to 120/80. If it is typically higher than 140/90, this may indicate some health concerns and require a trip to the doctor. A lower blood pressure reading usually means that your heart doesn't have to work very hard to pump the blood through your blood vessels.

I don't recommend those automatic blood pressure machines you find in drugstores or department stores; I have found that they give wildly varied blood pressure readings within the space of a few minutes, so I can't bring myself to trust them. You can ask your doctor, nurse, or qualified personal trainer at your gym to take your blood pressure. Or look for a clinic, health fair, or free medical screening at work or in your community.

Figuring Out Your Body Weight and Body Composition

This next group of tests helps make sense of your body weight and what it consists of. You may be amazed at how many ways you can measure your body. Consider all these measurements together to determine whether you are at your optimal weight and body composition.

Measuring your body weight

Measure your body weight on an accurate scale and record to the nearest half pound. Record your weight in Table 1-1. It's probably most accurate to weigh yourself in the nude because the weight of clothing and shoes can vary a great deal, depending upon your outfit. When you reweigh, try to do so at approximately the same time of day. Your weight can change by as much as five pounds during the course of a day. Don't weigh yourself more than once a week.

The weight you see on the scale tells you how many pounds you are — but not much else. Even those height/weight tables developed by insurance companies don't really give you much usable or accurate information. Neither the scale nor those charts tell you what your pounds are made of.

I used to work with three women who each weighed 130 pounds and who ranged from 5 feet 6 inches to 5 feet 11 inches in height. One of them was a muscular, body-building type, another was a lithe dancer, and the third was a triathlete with a little extra padding of fat which probably contributed to her success in swim events. According to the scale, all three women were very similar. However, looking at them side by side, you really get a sense that scale weight alone does not tell the entire story.

Don't weigh yourself — or at least limit the number of times you do so — if the numbers on the scale upset you. I personally never weigh myself and haven't in nearly ten years. I go by my clothing size and my body composition numbers.

Taking measurements of your body

Use your tape measure to make the following measurements to the nearest quarter inch. Take all measurements on the right side of your body. If you want, you can have a person whom you trust to keep your secrets help you take these measurements. Record the results in Table 1-1.

- ✔ **Upper arm:** Measure the largest part of your upper arm.
- ✔ **Chest:** Measure across your back and to the front, across the center of your chest.
- ✔ **Waist:** Measure the narrowest part of your torso above the belly button and below your chest.
- ✔ **Hips:** With your legs together, measure your hips and buttocks across the widest point.
- ✔ **Thigh:** Measure the widest circumference of your upper leg.
- ✔ **Calf:** Measure the widest circumference of your lower leg.

There are no "good" measurements or "bad" measurements. Measurements are more useful than straight scale weight for tracking changes because they indicate subtle improvements in your body composition. You may not have dropped a pound according to your bathroom scale, but you may have lost several inches on your thighs and hips.

Determining your body mass index

Body mass index (BMI) is a way of relating your height and weight to determine how fat you are.

You can figure out your BMI on your own, but you may need a calculator to perform these four easy mathematical steps. Take a deep breath — it's only arithmetic.

1. **Divide your body weight by 2.2.**

   For a 110-pound person, the calculation looks like this: 110 ÷ 2.2 = 50.

2. **Measure your height in inches and divide it by 39.4.**

   So, for instance, if you are 5 feet tall, that means you are 60 inches tall. 60 ÷ 39.4 = 1.5.

3. **Multiply your answer to Step 2 by itself.**

   For example, 1.5 x 1.5 = 2.3.

4. **Finally, take the number you arrived at in Step 1 and divide it by the number you arrived at in Step 3. Record your results in Table 1-1.**

   Your final number is an estimation of your BMI. To carry our example through, 50 ÷ 2.3 = 22. This means your BMI is approximately 22.

What does your final number mean? In 1999, the National Institutes of Health (NIH) issued the following BMI guidelines:

- ✔ **BMI of 18.5 or below:** You're considered underweight.
- ✔ **BMI between 18.5 and 24.9:** You're in the healthy range.
- ✔ **BMI between 25 and 29.9:** You're considered overweight.
- ✔ **BMI of 30 or greater:** You're considered obese.

BMI is a good though not perfect guide for determining whether you may need to lose or gain weight. For example, BMI measurements for extremely muscular athletes or pregnant women are not very accurate indicators. And, if your BMI is between 25 and 29, you shouldn't necessarily freak out about your weight. You must also consider other health factors — such as high blood pressure, whether you exercise, your smoking habits, and your family history of developing heart disease — to decide whether you need to drop a few pounds.

For those who fall within that 25 to 29 range, the NIH also recommends looking at your waist measurement. Men with a waist measurement greater than 40 and women with a waist measurement greater than 35 have a greater risk of developing heart disease than those with smaller waist measurements; if you fall into this category, you need to seriously consider losing weight for health reasons.

Measuring your waist-to-hip ratio

To determine this number, you can perform one simple mathematical step: Divide your waist measurement by your hip measurement. This number equals your waist-to-hip ratio. Here's a sample calculation to show you how easy it is.

If your waist measurement is 30 and your hip measurement is 36, you divide 30 by 36. 30 ÷ 36 = 0.83 for a waist-to-hip ratio of 0.83.

Men with a waist-to-hip ratio greater than 1 have a higher health risk. Women with a waist-to-hip ratio greater than 0.85 have a higher health risk.

If your ratio falls above these recommended numbers, you need to seriously consider losing weight. However, remember to take into account your scores for BMI and body fat percentage to help you make that decision.

Figuring out your body fat percentage

For this test, you need your hip measurement and your height in inches. Refer to the body fat chart in Figure 1-1. Place your tape measure or a ruler on the chart in a straight line between your hip measurement and your height. Draw a straight line between the two points with your pencil or pen. Your estimated body fat is the point where the line crosses the "percent fat" scale in the center. Record this number in Table 1-1 at the end of this chapter.

Your body fat percentage is an estimate of how much of your weight is fat and how much of it is lean body tissue, such as muscle, organs, and bones. If you determined from the chart in Figure 1-1 that your body fat is 20 percent, this means that an estimated 20 percent of your scale weight is fat.

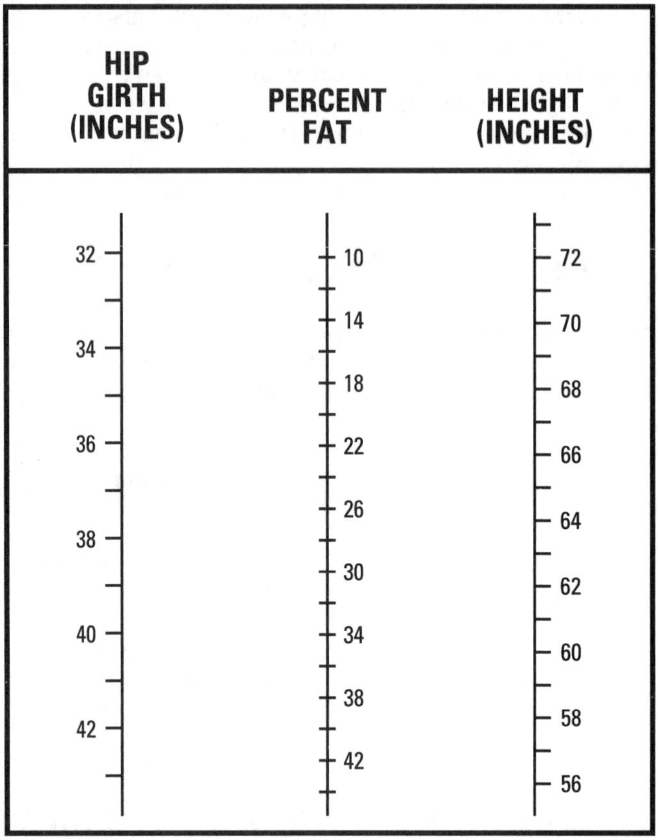

HIP GIRTH (INCHES)	PERCENT FAT	HEIGHT (INCHES)
32	10	72
	14	70
34	18	68
36	22	66
	26	64
38	30	62
40	34	60
	38	58
42	42	56

Figure 1-1: This chart can help you determine your percentage of body fat.

Human Kinetics Publishers, Inc.
Sensible Fitness, 2nd Edition
Jack Wilmove, Ph.D. CR-1986

Most fitness and medical experts consider body fat percentage a more accurate assessment of how fat you are than scale weight alone. However, experts have a wide range of opinions on what numbers are considered optimal. I take a conservative approach:

- ✔ **Men:** 12 to 20 percent body fat is considered optimal.
- ✔ **Women:** 16 to 26 percent body fat is considered optimal.

But just what does "optimal" mean? If you fall with the optimal range for your sex, you can be reasonably sure you're not overweight. However, this does not mean that you are thin or that you shouldn't consider losing weight. You must take into account all of the other body composition parameters that I discuss in this chapter to make that determination.

Women in particular need to be concerned with falling below optimal body fat ranges. With a body fat percentage of less than 10 percent, women can often have difficulty menstruating and are at higher risk for developing osteoporosis and other bone-degenerative diseases.

I think body fat percentage is best used as a guide to progress. When you take a body fat measurement a few months after you've been walking on a regular basis, it will more than likely go down. Because you have measured it at the starting point, you have a guidepost to compare to future measurements.

The chart method of body fat percentage measurement is a reasonably accurate way to get an estimate of body fat. If you have your body fat measured at your gym or doctor's office, the person measuring typically uses skin calipers or a bioelectrical impedance machine to do the estimation. The skin caliper method involves pinching various parts of your body with a giant tweezerlike device; the bioelectrical impedance method involves attaching small electrodes to one or more of your limbs. As long as trained and experienced professionals perform these tests, they can be extremely accurate. If you have a chance to get your body fat measured by a professional, I strongly recommend that you do so.

Measuring Your Strength and Flexibility

Lower body muscles provide most of the strength and power you need for walking, but that doesn't mean that the upper and middle body don't play their part. You will be a better walker if every muscle in your body is strong and ready to carry its share of the workload.

The following tests measure the *muscular endurance* of various areas of your body. Muscular endurance is a measure of how many times you can move a weight or perform an exercise when you're not pushing the heaviest load possible. However, I refer to the tests in this section as strength tests because this is how people talk in everyday life.

Taking stock of your upper body

One simple way to get a gauge of upper body strength is by doing a push-up test. Women should test their strength with a non-military push-up: Lie on your stomach on your mat or carpet with your palms flat on the floor just in front of your shoulders. Bend your knees so that your feet and lower legs are up off the floor. Now push yourself upward by straightening your arms and then bend your arms to lower yourself back down again. Only lower until your upper arms are parallel with the floor; keep your head and neck up and in line with the rest of your spine. Men should do regular "military-style" pushups in which they are balanced on their palms and toes. Do as many repetitions as you can without stopping.

Skip this test if you're prone to shoulder or neck problems. If you feel sharp pain in any of your joints as you do the test, stop.

This test is a gauge of how strong your chest, shoulders, and arm muscles are. These muscles are used in walking for a powerful arm swing.

How many push-ups can you do? Here's what your answer means:

- ✔ If you can do fewer than 11 repetitions, you are below average for upper body strength.
- ✔ If you do between 12 and 22 repetitions, you are average for upper body strength.
- ✔ If you do more than 22 repetitions, you are above average for upper body strength.

Measuring the strength of your middle body

The sit-up test is a good way to measure middle body strength. Get your stopwatch. Lie on your back with your feet about hip-width apart. Place your hands behind your head or across your chest, whichever way is more comfortable. Ask someone to hold your feet to keep them stable. Do as many sit-ups as you can in 1 minute. Count only full repetitions where your shoulder blade touches the floor when you're down and your knees touch your chest when you're up.

Don't arch your back or pull on your neck. Discontinue the test if you feel sharp pains in your neck or lower back. Don't even attempt it if you have a history of lower back or neck discomfort.

You're measuring a combination of abdominal, lower back, and hip flexor strength with this test. If you want to isolate your abdominal strength, you can perform a crunch test. Crunch tests are more difficult to set up and they're easier to cheat at, so I think they're best administered by a professional. If you have no back or neck problems, the sit-up test is safe and gives you some good information about your middle body strength.

How many sit-ups did you do? Here's what your answer means:

✔ If you can do no more than 20 repetitions, your middle body strength is below average.

✔ If you can do between 21 and 30 repetitions, your middle body strength is average.

✔ If you can do over 31 repetitions, your middle body strength is above average.

Seeing how strong your lower body is

The wall sit test helps you quantify your lower body strength. Get your stopwatch and stand about 2 feet away from a wall with your back pressed firmly against it. Keeping your feet flat on the floor, slide down the wall and bend your knees until you are in a seated position with your thighs parallel to the floor. Time how long you can hold this wall sit position.

If you have high blood pressure or bad knees, skip this test. If your knees begin to ache while you are in the wall sit position, stop.

The wall sit measures your buttocks and thigh strength. These are your powerhouse muscles used for walking.

How long can you hold the wall sit position? Here's what your answer means:

✔ If you can hold the wall sit position for no more than 30 seconds, your lower body strength is below average.

✔ If you hold the wall sit position for between 31 and 60 seconds, your lower body strength is average.

✔ If you hold the wall sit position for longer than 61 seconds, your lower body strength is above average.

Figuring Out Your Flexibility

Flexibility is an important measure for walkers. Lower body flexibility is the key to how long and smooth your stride is. You can take literally hundreds of flexibility tests, and nearly all can give you important information. In this section, I recommend three flexibility tests that I think give particularly useful feedback to walkers. If you hire a trainer who asks you to perform flexibility tests in addition to these, so much the better.

Determining the flexibility of your ankles

Sit on your mat or the floor with your legs straight out in front of you so that you are looking at your feet straight on. Point and flex your right foot and then point and flex your left foot. Note how far your can flex and point each of your feet.

This test is a measure of ankle flexibility. Ankle flexibility is important so that you get an adequate push-off when you walk. Here's what the results of this test mean:

- ✔ You should be able to *point* your foot away from you so that it is at least in line with your ankle. If you can't, you have below-average ankle flexibility.

- ✔ You should be able to *flex* your foot toward you so that it is beyond perpendicular with the floor. If you can't, you have below-average ankle flexibility.

Looking at lower back and hamstring flexibility

With your legs a few inches apart, bend over and touch your toes.

If you have a bad lower back, do not do this test. If, as you are bending over, your back hurts, discontinue the test.

The toe touch test measures lower back and hamstring flexibility. You may encounter other, more sophisticated, lower back and hamstring flexibility tests, but this one is the simplest. Here's what your performance on the toe touch test means:

- ✔ If you can't touch your toes, you have below-average lower back and hamstring flexibility.

- ✔ If you can touch your toes but only with considerable effort and/or slight discomfort, you have average lower back and hamstring flexibility.

- ✔ If you can easily touch your toes, you have above-average lower back and hamstring flexibility.

Determining your hip flexor flexibility

Lie on your back on your mat. Bend your right knee into your chest while keeping your left leg straight and note how easy it is to keep your left leg completely flat along the floor. Then do the same with your left leg.

How easily you can keep your opposite leg on the floor tells you how flexible the muscles in the front of your hips are. The flexibility of these muscles, called the *hip flexors,* is essential for a nice, long walking stride. If your hip flexors are tight, you may experience back pain as you walk. Here's what your performance on this test means:

✔ If you can't keep your straight leg completely on the floor, you have below-average hip flexor flexibility.

✔ If you can keep your opposite thigh on the floor but it's a little difficult to do so, you have average hip flexor flexibility.

✔ If you have no trouble keeping your opposite thigh on the floor, you have above-average hip flexor flexibility.

Taking a Look at Your Walking Endurance

Your endurance, stamina, or aerobic fitness can be gauged on a bike, stair climber, or treadmill. The best, most accurate way to assess this fitness parameter is with a test that most closely mirrors your primary activity, so I suggest an evaluation specifically designed for walkers. Once again, several other well-known walking tests can give you equally accurate results.

As a walker, you can test yourself on a bike or by some means other than walking. There's a certain amount of crossover of aerobic benefits from one type of aerobic activity to another. You may not do as well on a bike test if your main workout consists of walking, but you'll certainly do better than someone who doesn't exercise at all.

To do this test, you need a precisely measured 1-mile route that is as flat as possible. You can measure a course around your neighborhood by driving the distance in your car or, better yet, go to a track: The standard running track is a measured ¼ mile around. If you choose to do this test on a track, go during a time when it's not too crowded and use the inside lane. Here's how to do the test:

1. **Warm up with 5 minutes of easy walking.**

2. **Perform a few minutes of stretching and limbering up exercises.**

3. **Grab your stopwatch and start your timer.**

4. **Walk 1 mile (four times around the track) at a brisk, steady pace.**

   You should feel like you're pushing yourself reasonably hard but not so hard that you're unable to finish the mile. (If you can't complete the mile, that's okay. The fact that you can't tells you a lot about your fitness starting point.)

5. **When you reach 1 mile, stop your timer, and cool down for 5 minutes or so by walking at a slow, easy pace.**

   You can follow this cool-down walk with an easy stretch.

Compare your walking time with the results chart below.

Fitness level	Men	Women
Below average	Couldn't finish	Couldn't finish
Below average	15 minutes, 38 seconds or longer	16 minutes, 40 seconds or longer
Average	Between 12 minutes, 42 seconds and 15 minutes, 37 seconds	Between 13 minutes, 42 seconds and 16 minutes, 39 seconds
Above average	Less than 12 minutes, 42 seconds	Less than 13 minutes, 42 seconds

Using Your Results

After you complete all the fitness assessments in this chapter, don't just write them in your personal testing scorecard in Table 1-1 and close the book! Your results are the foundation of your walking program. Along with the information from the next chapter, you can use them to help set some pinpointed, detailed goals.

You shouldn't just test yourself once and leave it at that either. I recommend retesting yourself every three months or so and comparing the results to your previous test. There is nothing more motivating than seeing how far you've come since the beginning. If you don't want to do each and every test over again, just do the ones with the results that motivate you. I don't recommend retesting yourself more often than every three months because the body typically doesn't make changes that quickly. I do recommend doing a full retest at least once a year.

Table 1-1	Personal Testing Scorecard						
Subject of measurement	*First test*	*Three months*	*Six months*	*Nine months*	*One year*	*Optimal measurement*	
Resting and baseline parameters							
Resting heart rate						60–90 beats per minute (bpm)	
Resting blood pressure						120/80	
Body weight						Dependent upon gender and height	
Measurements (to the nearest ¼ inch)							
Right upper arm							
Chest							
Waist							
Hips							
Right thigh							
Right calf							
Body composition							
BMI						18.5–24.9	
Waist-to-hip ratio						Men = less than 1.0; Women = less than 0.85	
Body fat percentage						Men = 12-20 percent; Women = 16 to 26 percent	

(continued)

Table 1-1 _(continued)_

Strength	
Push-up	Greater than 22
Sit-up	Greater than 31
Wall sit	Greater than 61
Other	
Flexibility	
Ankle	Above average
Lower back and hamstring	Above average
Hip flexor	Above average
Other	
Endurance	
Walking endurance	Men = 1 mile in less than 12:42; Women = 1 mile in less than 13:42
Other	

Chapter 2

Going for Your Personal Gold

1 was developing a new program for a client, and, as I typically do, I asked her about her workout goals. "I don't know," she said, "I guess I want to lose weight and get in shape."

Her reply is probably the most common answer I get when I ask about goal setting — and I believe that this response is one of the main reasons so many fitness programs fall flat.

Embarking on a fitness routine is a major undertaking just like any other big project. You wouldn't build a house without a blueprint, and you wouldn't start a business without a detailed business plan. So why would you begin something as important as a fitness program without knowing where to start, where you're headed, and how you're going to get from start to finish?

In my experience as a personal trainer and exercise physiologist, I have come to believe that goal setting is an important and necessary process if you are truly serious about succeeding in your fitness program. In many ways, this goal-setting process is the defining moment of your walking program.

One reason people don't spend more time on goal setting is because they don't understand what constitutes a good goal. In this chapter, you find out how to set some definitive walking and fitness goals. I also offer guidelines for reaching and reevaluating those objectives.

Looking at the Six Essential Characteristics of Goals

Good fitness goals must possess six definite characteristics, outlined in the following sections. All six characteristics are equally important. Review your goals frequently to make sure that they meet these criteria.

Goals are specific

The problem with general goal statements like "I want to lose weight" or "I want to get in shape" is that they don't really mean anything specific. They don't tell you where you're starting from or what you ultimately hope to attain. How much weight do you want to lose? How "in shape" do you want to be?

Take the general statement "I want to lose weight" as an example. To hone this into a more specific goal, take a look at your starting point. The first thing you may want to do is change your thinking from "scale weight" to "body fat percentage" because body fat percentage is really a better measure of optimal weight and body size. (Turn to Chapter 1 and the sidebar "Translating your body-fat percentage into pounds," later in this chapter, for more information on body fat percentage.) For example, say that your body fat is now 30 percent. This piece of information instantly makes your goals unambiguous. Because you know that a generally accepted healthy level of body fat is 16 to 26 percent for a woman and 12 to 20 percent for a man, your aim becomes to lose at least 4 percent of body fat if you're a woman and at least 10 percent if you're a man, in order to fall within that range.

Using your body fat percentage is one way to specify clear goals. Another way is to point yourself toward a specific event, for example a 10K walk, that's coming up in a few months. Your goal may be to finish this event, or if you're more competitively minded, your goal can be to finish the event in less than 90 minutes. Both of these goals are specific enough to be meaningful because they are definitive aspirations. They also take into account your starting point, providing that you've evaluated how far and how fast you can walk right now.

Goals are realistic

I once received an e-mail from a singer who had just been signed to perform at an important engagement that was scheduled to take place the following day. She wanted to know how she could lose 15 pounds by the next night so that she could fit into the dress she had bought for the occasion. I told her to buy a new dress. Her goal was simply not realistically achievable — and, as I point out later in this chapter, it wasn't safe.

Translating your body fat percentage into pounds

Body fat is a more accurate measure of how "fat" you are than scale weight because it tells you how much of your weight is fat and how much of it is muscle or lean body mass. Still, if you're trying to lose weight, you may find it motivating to equate a drop in body fat percentage points with weight loss. Follow these four steps to make this translation:

1. **Multiply your current weight times your current body fat percentage.**

   To determine your percentage of Body Fat, flip to Chapter 1

2. **Subtract this number from your current body weight.**

3. **Subtract your target body fat percentage from 1.**

4. **Divide the number you got in Step 2 by the number you got in Step 3.**

This is the number of pounds you need to drop in order to achieve your goal body fat percentage.

Here's an example. Say that you now weigh 150 pounds, your current body fat percentage is 30 percent, and your target body fat percentage is 26 percent.

1. Multiply your current body weight by your current body fat percentage: $150 \times 0.30 = 45$. This number represents how much of your current weight is fat weight.

2. Subtract your fat weight from your current weight: $150 - 45 = 105$. This number represents your lean body weight.

3. Subtract 0.26 (your target body fat percentage) from 1. This equals 0.74.

4. Divide 105 by 0.74 to get 142 pounds, your target weight for a body fat percentage of 26 percent.

Achieving your goals can be a rewarding challenge. Not all of us have the capacity to climb to the top of Mount Everest or become an Olympic-level race walker. Strive for realistic and attainable goals. Don't aim so low that you find no glory in reaching your objectives, but neither do you want to strive for something that's completely, impossibly out of your reach.

Goals are adaptable

Revisit your objectives often in order to reassess and fine-tune them. For example, say that your original goal was to walk 3 miles, three times a week. But after a month or so of striving toward this aim, you find that your 3-mile walks take more than 45 minutes to complete and you simply don't have the time to do this. Instead of abandoning the goal and giving up walking altogether — as people so often do — adapt it to make it work. You may decide to rethink your goals based on time rather than distance. Or you may decide to spread your mileage goals out over 5 days rather than 3.

Be creative. You can adapt just about any goal to make it fit if you use your imagination.

Goals are healthy

A big reason the woman who wanted to drop several dress sizes in a day was barking up the wrong tree was that she was attempting to do something unhealthy, unrealistic, and dangerous to her body. I see this sort of thing all the time.

Quite often, unhealthy fitness goals revolve around weight loss or body shaping. Clients frequently give me a specific number they would like to see registered on the bathroom scale. When I ask why, the reasoning they offer is usually along the lines of "Because that's what I weighed in the eighth grade," or "Because I've always thought it would be nice to weigh so little." Many times their way of thinking is based upon irrational, destructive beliefs about themselves and their ideas of what their body should look like. Ultimately, this unhealthy approach leads some people into eating disorders like anorexia and bulimia.

Some goals are psychologically as well as physically unhealthy. I can't tell you how many times a client has plunked down a picture of Cindy Crawford or Tyra Banks in front of me and declared, "That's what I want you to make me look like!" Well, if you're 5-feet-1 with a curvy build, no amount of training in the world is going to turn you into a supermodel. It's very discouraging and psychologically damaging to think otherwise. That doesn't mean that you can't strive to look your best — but if you hold the view that an unattainable image is the only acceptable result, you're doomed to feel like a failure.

I want to dissuade you from this sort of ingrained, unhealthy thinking. Focus on the healthy fitness and weight guidelines set forth by various organizations including the American College of Sports Medicine and the American Council on Exercise and focus on being the best you can be without comparing yourself to anyone else. You can find contact information for these organizations in the appendix.

Goals are motivating

What gets you excited about your workouts? Is it that you can walk farther than the week before? Or perhaps the fact that you've trimmed an inch and a half from your waistline? Choose goals and objectives that make you look forward to your workouts. If they don't, reevaluate immediately. Having the most sensible goals in the world doesn't mean anything if they don't motivate you.

I have a client whose goal is to marry a hunk. She was very up front about this when she started working out in one of our gyms a few years back. She wanted to know the best times to work out and the best machines to frequent to meet eligible men.

Okay, so finding a husband isn't a fitness goal. But it's kept her working out on a regular basis for the past few years — and I've even managed to sneak a few fitness goals into her dream wedding plans. Although she hasn't snagged Mr. Right by walking on the treadmill four times a week and pumping iron in the free-weight room, she has never looked better and usually has a date on Friday nights. Whatever motivates *you* is what matters!

Goals are personal

Don't try to achieve something because your friend or your husband wants you to do it. Whether your objectives are related to health, athletics, or aesthetics, make them personal and meaningful to *you*.

Understanding the Different Types of Goals

Effective goal setting takes some forethought. For a goal to be truly meaningful, it needs to be carefully planned like an important event or the building of a house. When I do goal setting for myself or clients, I often take a single goal and look at it from several different angles.

Ultimate goals

Think of your ultimate goal as the big accomplishment, the thing you hope to achieve in the long run. In fact, you can also refer to your ultimate goals as your long-term goal.

ANECDOTE

Your ultimate goals typically take 2 to 12 months to achieve. One of my clients, Dutch, had the ultimate goal of trekking up to the base camp of Mount McKinley, one of the highest mountains in North America (base camp is the first significant stop on the way to the peak). He began his quest about a year before his planned trip. After we defined his ultimate goal carefully and in detail, we laid out an entire year's worth of workouts designed to help him achieve his ambition. Every day Dutch came in for his workout. Every day he visualized himself reaching Mount McKinley's base camp. This ultimate goal kept him motivated for the entire year. When he finally took that last step into base camp, he told me it was one of the most satisfying moments of his life. By the way, he was 65 years old at the time.

Your ultimate goal doesn't have to be something as monumental as climbing a mountain. Being able to walk the entire perimeter of the local park can be an ultimate goal that's just as satisfying and important. Some general examples of ultimate goals include, but aren't limited to, the following:

- ✔ Being able to walk a certain distance
- ✔ Being able to walk a certain speed
- ✔ Improving upon your evaluation results from Chapter 1
- ✔ Training for an event
- ✔ Improving your appearance
- ✔ Improving your health

Fine-tuned goals

Fine-tuned goals are simply a more detailed description of your ultimate goals. For instance, when Dutch and I looked at Dutch's ultimate goal of climbing to base camp (see the "Ultimate goals" section, earlier in this chapter), we researched how far he would have to walk, the steepness of the slopes he would encounter, and how heavy a knapsack he would have to carry. We designed his program with these factors into mind.

Your fine-tuned goals outline all the details you need to consider in order to reach your goals. You can use these fine-tuned goals to help lay out your program. Some things to consider when honing your fine-tuned goals include the following:

- ✔ Distance
- ✔ Speed
- ✔ Intensity
- ✔ Necessary skills
- ✔ Muscles being used

Stepping-stone goals

Having an ultimate goal that is a long way off can be discouraging. Having some shorter-term goals keeps you going from day to day. For this reason, it's important to have stepping-stone goals.

Stepping-stone goals simply break up your ultimate goals into smaller time-frames. For instance, if your ultimate goal is to walk a 5-mile loop around your neighborhood and you can only walk 1 mile right now, you may aim to walk a distance of 1.5 miles per workout next week, 1.75 miles per workout the week after that, and 2 miles per workout the week after that. By breaking up your ultimate goal into small, easily achievable, weekly goals, you set yourself up for victory time and time again. It also helps you stay focused on your ultimate goal because each stepping-stone goal that you can check off your list brings you one step closer to reaching your ultimate goal.

I recommend setting up stepping-stone goals that cover the following time-frames. You don't have to set goals for all these timeframes, but you may decide that it's worth the trouble to do so.

- ✔ **Daily goals:** What do you hope to accomplish today? It can be something as simple as going the whole day without eating chocolate or something as detailed as a thorough account of the workout you have planned. Daily goals are most effective when you're just beginning a workout program because they help you fine-tune your workout. They are also very useful if you're having trouble getting your butt off the couch.

- ✔ **Weekly goals:** Weekly goals are especially constructive for reevaluating targets like mileage and weight loss. Having a stepping-stone goal of a 1-pound weight loss per week can make your ultimate goal of a 30-pound weight loss become more manageable. Think about it: Weekly goals set you up for 52 small victories along the way every year. I like to reevaluate mileage goals on a weekly basis. For example, your stepping-stone goal for the coming week may be to increase your total mileage from 10 to 12 miles a week.

- ✔ **Monthly goals:** Monthly goals help you track trends in your workout patterns. You can simply multiply your daily and weekly goals to come up with what you'd like to shoot for over the course of the next 30 days. It's also a good idea to reevaluate your ultimate goal every month or so and do some tinkering if need be. You may decide that the goals you've outlined for yourself were too ambitious or that you can't reach them as quickly as you thought. Instead of being discouraged by this, take the time to redefine what you're trying to do. Reshape your goals and plans so that you can succeed.

Backup goals

Having goals that are adaptable means having backup goals — things you can shoot for if, for some reason, you aren't able to work toward your primary ultimate goals for a while. Backup goals keep you from getting discouraged or giving up.

For example, say that you've been working toward doing ten laps around the high school track in 40 minutes. You work your way up to six times around the track in 20 minutes . . . and then you pull a hamstring muscle and you're laid up for a couple of weeks. This sort of thing happens all the time and can be enough of a setback to make you abandon your walking program long after your muscle has healed.

In this case, you may have the backup goal of improving your upper body strength or decreasing fat in your diet. Instead of feeling disheartened by your injury, you can look at it as an opportunity to concentrate on something else for a while. Even if you aren't able to continue walking toward your ultimate goal right now, you don't need to feel that you've failed, because you're still making positive improvements in your health and fitness in the meantime.

The best backup goals are related to your ultimate goals or can contribute toward your ultimate goals in some way. Cutting fat from your diet, for example, may help you keep your weight down during a time when you are unable to burn off a lot of calories through exercise. It can prevent you from gaining weight and slowing you down when you can finally pick up where you left off. Here are some good general backup goals for walkers that you can tailor to your specific needs and preferences:

- ✔ Weight loss
- ✔ Improved appearance
- ✔ Increased energy
- ✔ Improved strength
- ✔ Improved flexibility
- ✔ Healthier diet
- ✔ Improvement in another activity like swimming or cycling
- ✔ Improved posture
- ✔ Enhanced self-esteem and self-confidence

Starting the Goal-Setting Process

Now that you know what constitutes a good goal to shoot for, you need a plan for how to reach it. I take a step-by-step approach to goal planning through the following sections.

Know your starting point

The first step in goal setting is determining your starting point by performing the series of fitness evaluations in Chapter 1. I cannot stress enough how important it is to perform some type of evaluation of where you are right now. You can't tell where you're going if you don't know where you've been. Your starting point lets you know, in no uncertain terms, what fitness parameters you need to work on.

Complete your personal testing scorecard (in Chapter 1) and note the aspects you can improve upon. Your goal-setting process can include strategies for making improvements in these areas. You may choose to highlight certain parameters over others as the focus of your program, but always strive for a balanced program. Even if you don't care that much about flexibility, for example, your overall program needs to include some stretching anyway. Why? Because all aspects of your health and fitness level are intertwined. If you pull a muscle because of lack of flexibility, you may be forced to take time off from your walking program, and that delay can prevent you from working toward your goals of weight loss and aerobic conditioning. Stretching also relieves and reduces the minor aches and pains associated with the early stages of walking. If you're more comfortable, you'll walk more.

Choose your ending point

Your ending point is your ultimate goal. Make sure that your ultimate goal has the six characteristics outlined earlier in this chapter.

Develop a plan

So how are you going to get from Point A to Point B? Actually, most of the rest of this book helps you answer this question. When planning your program, make sure that you include the types of activities and health changes that can help you work toward your ultimate goals and try to eliminate anything that may be counterproductive.

Develop your plan from the general to the specific. If you're trying to increase walking speed, you want to start out with the assumption that you have to practice walking faster. Then you can determine how many times and for how long you want to do speed training each week. You may also add weight loss, strength training, and flexibility work into your plan because these are goals that can help you get faster.

Planning successful workouts can be confusing if you don't know enough about what sorts of activities will help you get to where you want to go. This book helps you develop your plans. It also provides sample plans for you to follow. You can discover how to outline an accurate and successful walking program that is specifically tailored to you by reading Chapters 7 through 10. Additionally, these chapters offer tips on where to begin based on your current fitness level.

Write it down

Write everything down — all of your ultimate goals, your fine-tuned goals, your stepping-stone goals, and your backup goals. Tack your goal sheet to the refrigerator or the bathroom mirror and refer to it frequently so that you always have your eye on the prize. You can use the goal-setting worksheet at the end of this chapter for this purpose.

Write down your detailed plans as well. You can use this as a sort of checklist or blueprint for your workouts. I also strongly recommend keeping a workout diary, which includes the details of your workouts and diet (use the Walker's Log in this chapter).

Keeping a daily workout diary or journal is effective because it gives you a record to analyze long-term trends and it helps keep you honest. It helps you determine what you're doing wrong and what you're doing right. If you aren't making any progress, looking back through your log may tell you why. Perhaps you aren't working out as often as you thought you were, or perhaps you're eating more calories than you realized.

Many of my clients tell me that keeping a workout and diet diary is the best weight loss aid they've ever used. No one wants to write down that they've eaten a whole bag of cookies! I personally would skip eating them just so I wouldn't have to write that fact down on a piece of paper in permanent ink. And, on a positive note, writing down really great workouts or particularly successful eating habits is very satisfying.

Reevaluate

Reassess your goals from time to time to make sure that they're still in line with what you hope to achieve. Reevaluating your goals is especially important after you have achieved your ultimate goal. Take the time to savor the moment and do a victory lap on the treadmill — but then plan another event, think up another accomplishment, and determine where you'd like to move beyond this point.

I know that goal setting seems like a lot of work. But I cannot stress enough the importance of going through this process. Think of the testing and goal-setting process as the framework on which you are going to base your entire walking program. These processes help keep you consistent and motivated.

Walker's Log

Day of week	Date	Hours/miles walked	Comments
Monday			
Tuesday			
Wednesday			
Thursday			
Friday			
Saturday			
Sunday			
Total weekly mileage/minutes			
Stretched (number of days)			
Lifted weights (number of days)			
Other fitness activities			
Injuries, illness			
Weight			
Goals for upcoming week			

Goal-Setting Worksheet

Write down your *starting point*.

Write down your *ultimate goal*.

Write down your *fine-tuned goals*.

Write down your *stepping-stone goals* in detail.

Write down at least three *backup goals*.

Write down your *general plan* for achieving your ultimate goal.

Break down your general goal achievement plan in detail:

Monthly plan:

Weekly plan:

Chapter 3

Getting in Gear

• •

In This Chapter

▶ Discovering everything you need to know about walking shoes

▶ Choosing the right walking socks

▶ Gearing up for heat and cold

▶ Selecting the right sports bra

▶ Picking out safety gear and carriers

• •

*I*f you have any friends who are avid cyclists, you're probably familiar with the term "gearhead." The term is appropriate, given the amount of gear a dedicated cyclist requires for a half-hour ride: padded shorts or tights, a shirt with large pockets in the back, shoes that clip into the pedals of the bike, cycling gloves, sunglasses or goggles, and a helmet. Even the food is technologically engineered: Bikers munch on specially formulated energy bars and drink concoctions from specially designed fluid-delivery systems stored in those big pockets in the backs of their shirts. I won't even detail all the technology that goes into the bike itself.

Don't misunderstand me. I'm not putting down cycling as a pastime. For those people who love the ritual of putting on all this gear and clothing, I say, "Go for it." But for the non-gearhead who wants a basic, unfettered workout, there's walking.

Walking requires little more than a good pair of walking shoes. The right pair of shoes helps prevent injury, improve your performance, and keep you comfortable for up to 1,000 miles. In this chapter, I tell you everything you need to know about walking shoes — where to buy, what to buy, and how to buy. I also tell you the best way to lace them up according to your foot type, and how to prevent foot problems.

I also talk about other walking gear in this chapter, like socks and water bottle carriers. Do you absolutely need a pair of socks designed for walking, or a pouch to hold your water bottle? No. Does having this extra equipment make you a better walker? Perhaps. You'll probably find that at least some of the other gear mentioned in this chapter will enhance your walking experience. Use the information in this chapter to decide what walking gear works for you. For gizmos and gadgets that help you burn more calories and use more muscles when you walk, turn to Chapter 18.

Putting Your Best Foot Forward

Remember those sneakers you used to wear as a kid? Well, put those out of your mind. Going into a store and asking to see sneakers is like asking which aisle the gramophones and eight-track tapes are in. Any sales clerk under age 30 is going to assume you have a weird accent and direct you toward the "Snickers" bars in the candy department. Nowadays the shoes you walk in are called athletic shoes or, more precisely, *walking shoes*.

The good news is that the name change has done walking shoes a world of good. They really are better than the canvas footwear you used to wear to run faster and jump higher. A lot of technology has gone into them that unequivocally helps you improve your performance and avert injury.

Before you go shoe shopping, take the time to educate yourself. "Walking shoe" isn't the only bit of jargon your salesperson is going to throw at you. For instance, she may ask whether you over-pronate or supinate. She'll want to know if you prefer a wider toe box, more padding in the toe box, and if you need a board-lasted or combination-lasted shoe. Sound complicated?

Not really. I cover all these terms in this chapter, and I promise that after you get the lingo down pat and find out how to evaluate your needs, purchasing the perfect pair of walking shoes is a cinch. Start by assessing your feet and how you use them.

Finding out about your feet

Before you walk into a shoe shop, find out what type of foot you have walking in there. To evaluate your foot type, follow these easy steps:

1. **Place two pieces of construction paper side by side on a hard floor or on any surface on which they don't wrinkle when you step on them.**

2. **Wet your feet and pat them just dry enough so that they still remain a little damp.**

3. **Walk across the two pieces of paper and look at the results.**

   If you leave a large surface area footprint on the paper, you are an *overpronator*. This means that you have flat feet with not much arch. Your feet tend to roll excessively *inward* as they hit the ground. (Almost everyone's feet roll inward to some degree.)

If you leave just the marks of your toes, the balls of your feet, and heels, you are a *supinator.* Supinators have high arches and tend to roll the feet *outward* after they hit the ground.

What if your feet don't seem to fit into either of these categories? That means they're probably neutral. Neutral feet leave a footprint somewhere in between the pronator and supinator, showing the heel, the ball of the foot, the toes, and the outer underside of the foot. If you leave this type of footprint, your feet don't roll excessively outward or inward.

Another way to tell what foot type you are is to look at a pair of old shoes. Place them next to each other on a tabletop and look at them from behind at eye level. If your shoes cave inward severely, you are most likely a pronator. If they cave outward, you're probably a supinator. If they're fairly upright or cave in slightly inward, you have a neutral foot.

Keep your foot type in mind when you shoe shop. Foot type, along with a few other factors, helps determine which walking shoe works best for you. And if you happen to be a pronator or a supinator, be sure to give that information to the salesperson at the store where you shop. He or she can guide you to specific shoes made for feet like yours.

Dissecting the anatomy of a walking shoe

You don't need to know a lot of jargon related to walking, and what little there is usually refers to the shoes. Every single feature on a walking shoe has a name and a purpose (see Figure 3-1). Some shoes have patented devices to serve one or another of these purposes, but the following features are common to all decent walking shoes:

- ✔ **Sockliner:** You sometimes hear this called the *insole*. This is the removable insert that fits snugly at the bottom of the inside of the shoe. It's usually made from molded polyurethane of EVA (ethyl vinyl acetate), a synthetic shock-absorbing material.

- ✔ **Midsole:** The cushioning material between the bottom of the shoe and the sockliner, the midsole is the usually white or gray strip you see on the outside. The bulk of the cushioning is located here. Walking shoe midsoles are thinner than running shoe midsoles to allow for the rolling motion of your foot as you move through your walking stride. They are firm but flexible and well padded throughout, but especially at the heel where your foot strikes the ground, and at the ball of the foot where you roll through to push off into the next step. The midsole is also where shoe manufacturers place motion control inserts, which are made of hard plastic or dense foam. These devices help control the degree to which your foot pronates.

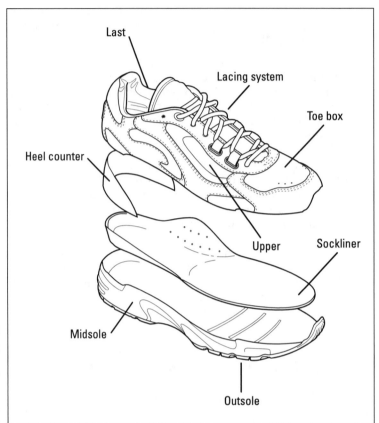

Last

Lacing system

Toe box

Heel counter

Upper

Sockliner

Midsole

Outsole

Figure 3-1:
The anatomy of a walking shoe.

The midsole is where the majority of the shoe's technology resides. Every company has a unique material or substance that it uses to provide cushioning and shock absorption. Nike, for instance, inserts little air pillows in the midsole. Reebok also uses air to provide cushioning but in a slightly different way: It runs a series of chambers through the midsole. When you strike down on your heel, the impact forces the air through the chambers and into the front of the shoe. By the time you roll through on to the ball of your foot, a cushion of air is there waiting for you. Other companies use gel or EVA.

✔ **Outsole:** Also referred to as the *outer sole,* the outsole is the bottom of the shoe, including the treads. It provides further cushioning, as well as traction. On walking shoes, the outsole should be firm and higher in the heel than under the ball of the foot. Outsoles are usually made from durable, carbon-based rubber. Stay away from leather soles — they're too slippery and usually mean that the shoe is not meant for athletic walking.

✔ **Heel counter:** A hard, molded plastic or cardboard structure that wraps around the heel, the heel counter is located on either the inside or outside of the shoe, depending on the model. The heel counter is the device that keeps the heel centered and stable as your foot strikes the ground. You can't always see the heel counter because it often resides between the lining of the shoe and the upper. If you're not sure what you're looking for, ask the salesperson about this feature.

✔ **Toe box:** This is the front part of the shoe that houses your toes. People with wide feet should seek out a shoe with a wide toe box; people with narrow feet should seek out a narrower toe box. The toe box should be wide enough to allow you to wiggle your toes comfortably and long enough so that a thumbnail sized space remains in front of your longest toe.

✔ **Upper:** The top part of the shoe, which is sewn or glued to the midsole. The upper is usually made of leather, nylon mesh, or some combination of both. I prefer nylon mesh uppers because they breathe better and your feet don't get all sweaty during your workout. Nylon mesh doesn't stretch out either, so your shoe stays the same size throughout its entire life span. Leather uppers are easier to keep clean, though.

✔ **Last:** In shoespeak, the *construction last* is the plastic, metal, or fiber mold around which the shoe is built. It determines the shape and fit of the shoe and also influences its flexibility and stability. There are three main last categories:

- **Board lasting:** A method of shoe construction that uses stiff materials, which makes for a more stable, rigid shoe. When you remove the sockliner insert and look at the inside bottom of a board-lasted shoe, you can see that the shoe has a cardboard insert around which the shoe is constructed.

- **Slip lasting:** A method of shoe construction that creates a more flexible shoe than board lasting. This type of construction is usually used to provide flexibility where the toes bend. When you remove the shoe insert and look at the inside bottom of a slip-lasted shoe, you can see that it is sewn together along the entire length of the cloth lining of the shoe; the stitching resembles a Frankenstein scar. Improvements in shoe design and technology have made slip-lasted shoes more stable than they used to be.

- **Combination lasting:** Combines the flexibility of slip lasting with the stiffness of board lasting. A shoe using combination lasting is glued together from the mid-foot back, and sewn together from the mid-foot forward.

✔ **Shoe shape:** Shoes come in all different shapes. You'll probably find that one shape roughly mirrors the shape of your foot and therefore will be the most comfortable. You can determine the shape of your shoe by turning it over and looking at the outline of the bottom of the shoe.

- **Straight:** Turn your shoe over and look at the outer sole. If it doesn't curve inward toward the big toe, it's straight.

- **Curved:** Turn your shoe over and look at the outer sole. If it curves inwards toward the big toe, it has a curved shape. There is also a semi-curved shape, which is a nice in-between option.

✔ **Lacing system:** You can't have just laces anymore; you have to have a system. The typical system consists of holes and D-rings. The D-rings allow for faster lacing, a better fit, and greater comfort. Some lacing systems also include a *stability strap* that runs from the midsole and connects with the lacing system. The purpose of the strap is to help keep your foot snugly in place, to support your arches, and to improve the fit of the shoe.

Laces themselves have also been souped up for the modern world. They are usually made of a synthetic blend rather than cotton so they last longer and stay tied. Really good laces have an oval shape with two seams situated opposite each other. Oval laces stay tied so you never have to worry about stopping in the middle of a walk for a shoelace that's flapping in the breeze.

Choosing the best shoe for you

A good pair of walking shoes runs you anywhere between $40 and $100. Price depends on brand, features, and style. After you find a pair you like, shop around for the best price. I highly recommend catalog and Internet shopping. The Road Runner Sports catalog in particular — also available on the Internet — offers competitive prices and a wide selection of both running and walking shoes. The catalog is available at www.roadrunnersports.com.

Walking shoes in general have good shock absorption in the heels and in the balls of the feet. They are a bit stiffer and more supportive than running shoes, although they have a very flexible forefoot (front page of the shoe) to allow for the natural bend of the foot. The midsoles are thinner than those of running shoes in order to accommodate the slower foot roll when you walk. They feature beveled, or slightly angled, heels to allow for a smooth heel-to-toe roll. Beyond these basic traits, look for a shoe that meets your needs in terms of foot type, injury patterns, mileage, speed, and walking surface, all of which are covered in the following sections.

Finding a shoe to match your foot type

Knowing your foot type and having a basic understanding of shoe terminology under your belt should help you determine the type of shoe that's best for you. Even before you put the shoe on your foot, you should be able to do a quick inspection and have an idea as to whether it's a good choice for you or not. Of course, you should always try on any shoe you buy for fit and comfort.

- ✔ **Pronators** should look for a shoe with a motion control device in the midsole. They also should look for a board-lasted, straight shoe, which provides support for the inside of the foot and thus prevents you from overusing the inside edge of your foot. Pronators should also look for a reinforced heel counter for control and stability. Sturdy uppers and stability straps can also help prevent inward roll. Shoes with too much padding can exaggerate pronation, so avoid them.

- ✔ **Supinators** should look for greater stability and a shoe whose outer sole, insole, and midsole are designed for extra shock absorbency. Slip-lasted, curved shoes are probably your best bet because supinators have such rigid feet. Buy shoes with reinforced material around the ankles and firm heel counters for maximum ankle and heel support. Extra cushioning under the ball of the foot helps increase comfort.

- ✔ Owners of **neutral feet** can wear just about any shoe and be ensured of proper support and comfort, but you may find that shoes that have a curved shape fit best. Even if your feet are neutral and you have no injury issues, don't skimp on the basic walking shoe features.

Taking note of injury patterns

Take stock in your usual points of injury — even if your walking routine didn't cause them. If you are prone to any sort of joint pain in your ankles, knees, hips, or lower back, look for a well-cushioned shoe that allows your foot to move naturally. Definitely make an effort to walk in walking shoes as opposed to dress shoes or running shoes.

Dress shoes, especially women's shoes with tall heels, change the entire alignment of your spine. They are often the culprit causing knee, back, and ankle pain. Obviously, sometimes women must wear dress shoes with heels, but try to keep those times to a minimum by slipping on your heels at the last minute and slipping them off your feet when appropriate.

Walking in running shoes forces your foot muscles to work much harder to keep your foot stable and to flex the foot. Also, the thicker midsoles make your foot smack down on the pavement. Over time, walking in running shoes may also exacerbate joint injuries, especially shin splints.

Chronic joint problems may have to be addressed with specially designed shoe inserts called *orthotics*. Orthotics help correct the way your foot hits the ground and thus relieve a lot of problems caused by the shocks that travel up through the joints as a result of faulty footfall.

Orthotics must be custom designed and crafted by a podiatrist or foot doctor. They can cost anywhere from $50 to $200 depending on the design and materials. Do not attempt to build your own orthotics. I have a client who went out and purchased several pairs of store-bought inserts, cut them up, and stacked them like blocks in his shoes. After a few days of walking around on these homegrown orthotics, he began complaining of knee and ankle pain. When he told me what he had done, I counseled him to remove the inserts from his shoes immediately.

Your feet support your entire body weight. If you do something to throw your feet off-kilter, you very often cause problems elsewhere in your body.

For those of you prone to friction injuries like corns, bunions, and blisters, look for shoes with a wide, roomy toe box. New Balance is one of the few athletic shoe companies that sells various widths from AAA to EEE. Many stores don't carry the full line of New Balance sizes, but many mail order catalogs do. You may want to experiment with walking sandals that leave your usual hot spots exposed and free from the friction-producing parts of the shoe, like the upper. Nike and Teva make very good walking sandals. Of course, sandals aren't always practical; you certainly can't walk through a snowdrift in them.

Keeping in mind mileage, speed, and walking surface

Walkers who average more than 30 miles a week and/or who walk for speed should look for *high-performance* walking shoes. Here's what to look for in a high-performance shoe:

- Light weight
- Lots of specialized, extra features to improve stability, cushioning, and shock absorption, like reinforced heel counters, stability straps, and high-tech midsole and insole materials
- Removable insoles with some arch support
- Cushioning that is firm and springy but not as wiggly as gelatin
- Extra cushioning, especially in the heel and ball of the foot
- Flexibility that matches the natural bend of the foot
- Sturdy uppers, usually made of nylon mesh
- D-ring lacing system that allows for variable lacing patterns, which means that the eyelets are situated at various distances from the center of the shoe

Most major brand walking shoes are high performance shoes. These brands include Nike, Reebok, Saucony, New Balance, Asics, and Adidas. Casual walkers can look at brands like Easy Spirit and Spenco. Though these latter two are perfectly fine shoes, I do not consider them high performance.

Lacing up right

Think you learned all you need to know about tying your shoelaces when you were 4 years old? Think again. There are many variations on the traditional crisscross lacing technique. Try one of the following lacing systems:

- If you have narrow feet, get shoes with a *variable lacing system.* A variable lacing system has two or three sets of eyelets located at different distances away from the center of the shoe. For a snugger fit in the heel, use only the set of eyelets farthest away from the center of the shoe *(see Figure A).*

- If you have very wide feet and a variable lacing system, pull the laces through the eyelets closest to the center of the shoe to create a little extra toe wiggle room (see Figure B).

- If you are blister-prone, lace up in a different way: Use the traditional crisscross method until you reach the second-to-last eyelet. Thread the lace through the last eyelet on the same side so that you create a loop on either side of the shoe. Then crisscross one lace end over pull an end through each loop (see Figure C). Tighten and tie. This helps keep your foot from sliding around as you walk.

- If you have high arches, thread your laces, pointing down, in the bottommost eyelets. Take the left lace and thread it through the third eyelet from the bottom on the left side. Thread the right lace through the second eyelet on the right side and then through the second eyelet on the left side. Return to the left lace and cross it over to the right side and thread it through the third eyelet on the right. Continue this pattern until you reach the top of the shoe and lace the last two eyelets up in a standard crisscross (see Figure D). This method helps your foot spread out evenly in the shoe to prevent pain in the arch and at the top of the foot. It may seem complicated, but after you read the directions a few times, you'll get the hang of it.

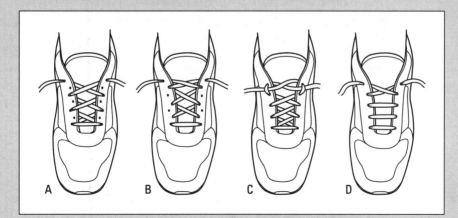

A   B   C   D

If you do most of your walking on trails or rocky, sloped, uneven terrain, a hiking shoe or boot is a must for traction and foot protection. Hiking shoes possess many of the same features as walking shoes, with a few notable differences: They have added heel and ankle support, sturdier soles and treads, and uppers made of leather. Nike and some of the other major shoe companies make excellent hiking shoes and boots; other companies, such as HighTec, Lowa, and Salomon, concentrate their footwear efforts solely on hiking boots. Companies like Rockport and Timberland also make "rugged walkers" that are specifically designed for trails and high mileage. I prefer the specialized brands because they cater to the features and comfort sought by serious hikers. They are more expensive though: Good hiking boots start at about $80 and can cost as much as $200.

Shopping for shoes

Now that you're armed with information about your foot type and shoe terminology, you can start shopping for walking shoes. The typical athletic shoe store has at least 8 to 30 styles of walking shoes to choose from. Give yourself at least an hour the first time you shop for walking shoes to make the perfect selection. Follow these suggestions and you can't go wrong.

- ✔ **Shop at a specialty store, rather than a department store, if possible.** This may cost you some extra bucks, but having a knowledgeable salesperson to guide you can mean the difference between a great purchase and getting stuck with unwearable clodhoppers. Later, when you become a more experienced shoe shopper, you can save up to 50 percent by shopping in a department store, by catalog, or on the Internet.

- ✔ **Write down all the information you discovered about your feet and your walking program.** If you have an old pair of walking shoes, bring them with you so you can show the salesperson your wear pattern. Take along the socks you usually wear, too, so that you can size your new shoes the way you'll actually be wearing them.

- ✔ **Examine each pair of shoes before you try them on.** Turn them over. Does the shape match your foot type? Does it have a good strong heel counter? Slip out the insert to discover what type of last the shoe is built on. Bend the shoes back and forth a few times. Are they flexible in the forefoot? (This shoe-testing process can make you feel like you're selecting the best melon at the supermarket.)

- ✔ **Put on both shoes and lace them up completely. Walk around the store for a few minutes to get the feel of the shoe.** Whenever possible, try them on a hard-surfaced floor. Paragon, a shoe and clothing store in New York, has a treadmill handy so that shoe buyers can test-drive their shoes at various speeds. Your primary concern should be comfort. If the shoes are not comfy from the second you put them on your feet, put them back in the box and try another pair. Do not buy a shoe with the plan of "breaking them in." Doing so is begging for the agony of the feet.

- ✔ **Be prepared to test several different shoe models.** Even if you like the first shoe you lace up, try at least two other models for comparison purposes. Don't be swayed by what your personal trainer or your hairdresser wears. Each person has unique walking shoe needs. One person's favorite shoe can turn another person's feet into road kill.

- ✔ **Always shop later in the day because your feet can swell up to half a size larger during the course of the day.** Shoes that fit in the morning may be too snug for afternoon workouts. Have the salesperson measure both of your feet each time you shop so that you can note any size changes. A shoe that fits well has about a thumbnail's space between your longest toe and the end of the toe box. Always accommodate your longest toe and your largest foot.

- ✔ **When you find a shoe you like, buy it and try it out for a few days.** If you absolutely love it after three workouts, go back and buy a couple pairs of the same shoe. Shoe companies have an annoying habit of phasing out and "upgrading" shoe models on a regular basis. If your shoe is discontinued, that's it. You have to start the whole selection process all over again. Shoe companies never revive discontinued models.

Shoe companies phase out older models for marketing purposes, but this policy can be very frustrating for those of us who are serious about our workout programs and have a loyalty toward a particular model. I used to wear Nike Air Zooms, a model I loved so much that I named my dog Zoomer in honor of it. After it was discontinued, I went so far as to call the manufacturer directly to buy up whatever stock was left. Inevitably, I wore out my last pair and had to find a new favorite shoe. Needless to say, if I got my dog today, he'd have a different name, probably 745, after my New Balance 745s.

Searching for a Good Sock

Don't go sockless when you walk. Socks absorb sweat and prevent friction between your feet and the inside of your shoe. Sockless walkers frequently complain of blisters, chafing, and athlete's foot. Their feet and shoes often smell bad, too.

Fortunately, you can leave most of the jargon and complex technology in the shoe department. Purchasing a walking sock is a much more straightforward task. I highly recommend testing out several different types of socks to see what type and brand you like best. You don't have to buy socks specifically designed for walking, but you should look for a few basic traits.

- ✔ **Socks that are thick, but not too thick, are your best bet.** Dress socks, nylons, and very thin socks don't prevent enough friction to be worn alone, although when worn under your main socks they can help keep your foot from rubbing against the inside of your shoe. Some socks have extra padding in the heel and forefoot. This extra padding is not essential, but some walkers like the extra cushiony feel.

- ✔ **Cheapo tube socks are also a no-no because they tend to bunch around your toes and lose shape very quickly.** They also hold sweat and heat up your feet, which can be uncomfortable, especially when you walk in hot weather.

- ✔ **Stick to synthetic fibers like acrylic and Dupont's CoolMax.** Though natural fibers like cotton and wool feel great at first, they lose their shape quickly and don't do a very good job of "wicking away" moisture.

- ✔ **Whatever sock you decide on, make sure that it doesn't bunch around the toes or gather at the heels.** This can cause blisters and hot spots.

- ✔ **Don't buy socks that are too small.** That's like wearing a shoe that's too small; it places too much pressure on the ends of your toes.

- ✔ **When your socks wear out, lose shape, or have holes in them, chuck them and buy new ones.**

I have done very well with socks made by a company called SmartWool. These socks are made of wool that has the feel of a natural fiber but behaves like a synthetic. SmartWool socks do a fantastic job of pulling sweat away from your feet and letting them breathe. The socks hold shape even when wet and even after numerous washings. They cost up to ten bucks a pair — a bit more than your average sock — but if you're going to splurge, this is a good purchase. Thorlo and Wigwam also make excellent athletic socks. If, in spite of my warning against wearing thin socks for walking, you like a thinner sock, try Defeet brand socks. Although they are on the thin side, they are well padded and do a good job of reducing friction.

Dressing Well for Walking

Many lifestyle walkers (see Chapter 7) walk in their regular clothes. There's nothing wrong with that so long as what you wear does not impede your movement. For instance, wearing a long, tight skirt that cuts your natural walking stride short isn't a good idea.

Comfort is the only real requirement your walking clothes need to meet. It's also nice if they reflect your personality.

When I lived in Brooklyn a few years back, my husband and I used to run over the Brooklyn Bridge to get to work in Manhattan every morning. We'd often see a group of about ten women walking into Brooklyn, all of them dressed in pink from head to toe — pink sweat suits, pink socks, pink sweatbands. Let me tell you, they were quite a sight. We looked forward to seeing "The Pink Gang," as we nicknamed them, striding in lockstep with purpose and determination.

As for fitness walkers, your clothes should be comfortable and nonrestrictive. Dress appropriately for the weather and situation, which, of course, changes with the temperature.

Knowing what to wear in warm weather

The right wardrobe can make warm-weather running more tolerable. A light-colored, loose *singlet* (mesh tank top) is best. In direct sunlight, provide your body with as much shade as possible — a light-colored cap with a rim, sunglasses, and of course, a liberal application of sunscreen. Wear shorts or short tights — this is strictly a matter of preference. Synthetic fibers designed to let moisture escape and evaporate quickly are the most comfortable. Clothes made from natural fibers, like cotton, feel cool and comfy when you first put them on, but after you start sweating, the fabric feels wet and clammy. If you like the feel of cotton against your skin, experiment with cotton synthetic blends. To complete your outfit, grab a water bottle or some sort of hydration system like a camelback water sack.

Knowing what to wear in cold weather

When dressing for winter walking, remember that three thin layers work better on the upper part of your body than one or two thick ones to keep you warm. Each layer traps air, which acts as an insulator to retain body heat.

The layer closest to your body serves as a *vapor transmission or moisture wicking* layer. That's just a fancy way of saying that it draws perspiration away from your skin. The best materials for the job are lightweight and synthetic. The middle "insulating" layer should consist of a sweater, sweatshirt, vest, or shell. It should be lightweight and unrestrictive so that it doesn't prevent you from moving naturally and generating your own body heat. Fabrics like Gore-Tex and Polar Guard work well. Natural fibers like wool are also excellent because they retain warmth even when wet. (By the way, cotton is a real no-no because it gets wet easily and stays wet. It loses shape, too.) The outermost, protective layer serves as a shield from wind and water; it should trap heat but also be breathable. A jacket, pullover, or windbreaker works well. Whatever material your outer layer is made from, just make sure that it is waterproof as opposed to water resistant. You don't want to find out the hard way that there's a significant difference between the two!

On the bottom half of your body, you can get away with one or two layers, depending on how cold it is and what type of precipitation is falling. I prefer Lycra tights because they fit snugly but don't restrict movement. But if you prefer sweats or wind pants, that's fine as long as they protect you sufficiently.

Accessorize with mittens and a hat. In general, mittens are preferable to gloves because they keep your hands warmer. I see many walkers with neck and face warmers, but I find them an annoyance. To keep my neck warm, I wear a turtleneck. On bright, sunny days, wear sunglasses and sunscreen; light reflecting off the snow can be just as strong and skin-damaging as the midsummer sun reflecting off the water. Don't forget to bring your water along, too.

Here's a good rule to follow for your winter workout wardrobe. Dress as if it's 10 degrees warmer that it really is. When you first start out, you'll be chilly, but after you get moving, you should feel just right. You can always stop and peel off a layer if you get too hot.

Shopping in Catalogs for Your Walking Gear

Plenty of catalogs cater to walkers and runners. You can often get good bargains when you shop by catalog or via the Internet. Personally, this is the only way I shop for my workout clothes. I have my favorite catalogs and I know which ones stock the stuff I like. These are three I recommend:

- **RaceReady:** Carries a wide variety of brightly colored walking clothes, from tights to shorts to fleeces. You can find every conceivable walking accessory in this catalog, plus a few you probably never even dreamed existed. Contact information: phone 800-537-6868 or Web site www.raceready.com.

- **Road Runner Sports:** Don't let the name fool you. This catalog has a great selection of both running and walking clothes. I always buy my tights from this catalog because it offers them in variable lengths. You can also access this catalog on the Internet. Road Runner delivers within two days and has a liberal return policy. I find the phone consultants helpful and knowledgeable as well. Contact information: phone 800-551-5558 or Web site www.roadrunnersports.com.

- **Title Nine:** This women's-only clothing catalog is a real discovery. It sells hard-to-find brands like Moving Comfort. I have a favorite windbreaker I bought from this catalog several years ago. The thing I love best about this jacket is the extra-long flap in the back that comes down and covers my butt. Contact information: phone 800-609-0092 or Web site thefolks@title9sports.com.

For Women Only

ANECDOTE

"Hi, people. I wonder if anyone can give me some suggestions for an embarrassing question that came up when I was walking the other day. I'm fairly busty (not huge, but a D cup), and even with a good-quality sports bra, I find I still get a lot of bounce — not just jiggling, but up-and-down, side-to-side bounce. It's mentally distracting and darned uncomfortable! I am looking forward to hearing from anyone who's got any ideas or suggestions!"

This is an actual question I received on my Fit By Friday Internet bulletin board located on the iVillage Web site, www.ivillage.com. It's not an uncommon question, and it's one that's close to many women's hearts — in more ways than one.

Choosing the right sports bra

Proper breast support is vital for physical, psychological, and emotional comfort. When your breasts bounce and move as you exercise, it can be painful. Bouncing can cause the small ligaments of the breasts (called Cooper's ligaments) to stretch. Over time, this stretching can lead to sagging. Additionally, bouncing can be distracting and make you feel self-conscious. Who needs to be more self-conscious when they're exercising?

Fortunately, finding a good bra is easier than it used to be. You have a couple different options to choose from.

Compression bras

The original type of sports bra parallels other types of body supports, like Ace bandages and jock straps. These are called *compression bras* because they press the breasts up against the chest as a single mass. These come in a "crop top" design with one large piece of material to hold your breasts in place. Larger-breasted women may experience discomfort with this type of bra because the breasts can still bounce around as a single unit.

Encapsulation bras

Larger-breasted women may find a newer type of sports bra, known as an *encapsulation bra,* helpful. Encapsulation bras hold each breast in a separate cup so they stay in place and don't press against each other. Many are sized like traditional bras up to size DD, whereas compression bras usually come in small, medium, and large.

Banish the bounce

Today's women exercisers take the existence of the sports bra for granted, but just 20 years ago, sports bras didn't exist. That was before a resourceful woman named Hinda Miller had a chance encounter with a jock strap.

As a medium-breasted runner who was tired of flimsy bras with straps that wouldn't stay put, Miller asked about a sports bra at a local lingerie shop. The saleswoman looked at her like she had just stepped off a spaceship from Mars. She complained to a friend who then pulled a jock strap out of the wash and declared, "Jock bra!" Miller knew she was onto something.

As it happened, Miller was also a costume designer. She and her partner fashioned the JogBra prototype in 1978 by sewing two jock straps together; samples of this prototype are on display at the Smithsonian Museum in Washington, D.C., and the Metropolitan Museum of Art in New York City. Today, most women who exercise wear some type of sports bra for comfort and safety. The sports bra industry is now a $30 million business. JogBra eventually became a division of the lingerie giant Playtex.

Buying and wearing your sports bra

Try both types of bras — compression and encapsulation — to see which one works best for you. When you try a sports bra on, raise your arms over your head. If the elastic band at the bottom rises up, the bra is not the size to give you enough support. Try the next size up. Also, jump around in the dressing room. If you feel the bounce there, you're definitely going to feel it when you go stepping out. And make sure that any bra you buy for exercising is at least 25 percent Lycra.

If all else fails and you can't find a bra that stops the bounce, here's a tip many large-breasted women have had success with: Wear two sports bras at once. Try a compression bra over an encapsulation bra, making sure that the straps cross differently around the back. The combination of the two types of bras creates an overlapping support and should keep things pretty still, though it may be a bit much in hot weather.

Some good brands to try include Lontex, Moving Comfort, Champion, Nike, and Danskin. Most cost $20 to $30 and are available in sports specialties stores. Try before you buy. When you find a brand and style you like, you can often find it at a steep discount in a clothing catalog.

Getting Hip with Reflective Gear and Carryalls

Many walkers have a need for things that make you stand out in the dark. Others like to carry their liquid and other items in a handy place.

Safety and reflective gear

Reflective gear is a must for anyone who walks when it's dark. There is no shortage of reflective products. You can spend hundreds of dollars for a full outfit that has reflective accents strategically placed for maximum visibility, or you can spend just a few bucks for sew-on or stick-on reflective patches that you place on the clothing yourself. However much you decide to spend, it's well worth it, especially if you walk anywhere near moving cars or bikes.

At a recent trade show, I counted over 100 reflective and lighted products. I saw everything from caps with built-in blinking lights, to glow-in-the-dark collars and leashes for dogs. I even saw a new brand of reflective paint that you brush onto your clothing and is good for up to 50 washes.

You don't need to spend big bucks on expensive reflective clothing if you don't want to. A good place to buy inexpensive reflector products is in a hunting shop or sporting goods store that specializes in outdoor sports, where you can find reflective vests like construction workers wear, and bright orange jackets like deer hunters wear. You can also find reflective tape and oversized buttons in a hardware store or big discount store. I once saw a walker who made a necklace out of the reflectors you stick on the back of bicycles. It looked a little strange, but it did the trick. I talk more about reflective gear in Chapter 18.

Carriers

You probably have to carry something with you, even on short walks. Your keys, a water bottle, some money — by the time you gather together everything you need, your hands are full, and you have to start stuffing things in pockets. You may want to think about purchasing some sort of pouch or carryall to keep your various sundries in one easy-to-reach place. You can choose from a wide variety of options.

✔ **Fanny pack:** These small oblong pouches clip on like a belt around your waist and are often called hipsters or fanny packs. Many are designed to carry your portable tape player as you exercise. I don't think you should be listening to headsets while you walk, unless you do your walking on a treadmill. It's not safe to tune out your surroundings in this manner. However, these pouches are the perfect size for carrying your keys, money, and a few other accessories.

Fanny packs generally cost from $10 to $25. They're made of neoprene or some other quick-dry material. Most of the ones I've seen fit around your waist: People either rest the pouch under their waist or turn it around so it rests just above the buttocks. I never could figure out which is proper protocol, though I suspect that one group secretly makes fun of the other. I recently saw a fanny pack that was designed to fit up high on the back and was secured by a strap that ran across the chest.

✔ **Water bottle holders:** This is simply a variation on the fanny pack. The typical configuration snuggles around your waist and has a pocket or two to hold your keys and money, and a large padded opening for your water bottle. Some models hold two water bottles, which is perfect if you're going to walk a long time in hot weather with little opportunity for a refill.

I know people who swear by these water bottle holders. I have never been able to get used to wearing one. The water bottle always jostles around — or so it seems to me. My husband usually accuses me of being like the Princess and the Pea when I complain about this.

If, like me, you're sensitive to weight around your waist, there are hand-held options and *liquidpacs,* water sacks that strap on to your back and have a long hoselike straw for you to sip through.

✔ **Key holders:** You have a couple of choices in key holders. You can buy nifty little pockets with a loop for your shoes. You thread the loop into your shoelaces to secure the pocket to your shoe. You can also find key holders built into the lining of some walking shorts. Key holders are usually just large enough to hold a key or two and perhaps some change. Even I can't complain that this little gadget distracts or annoys me in any way.

Chapter 4

Nutrition for Walkers on the Run

· ·

In This Chapter

▶ Understanding the basic fuel groups

▶ Looking at the food pyramid

▶ Discovering the ABCs of vitamins, minerals, and other nutritional considerations

▶ Knowing why you have to give up on dieting

▶ Eating well for walking performance

▶ Getting the scoop on fast food and junk food

· ·

*E*very day, one of my clients asks me whether she should buy some crazy diet book on the bestseller list or believe the outrageous nutritional claim she read about in a popular magazine. Lynn, a client who has been working out with me for about five years, once announced that she was going on a high-protein diet. She wanted to give up all carbohydrates, including whole grains, pasta, and rice, because she read that they make you fat. Mind you, Lynn wants to run a marathon. She is training very hard, running and walking as many as 40 miles a week.

How many nutty, too-good-to-be-true nutritional theories have you heard or read about lately? How many have you believed? How many have you tried? How many have worked? On the surface, these theories appear perfectly credible — often backed up by seemingly respectable studies, reliable scientific information, and glowing testimonials. And yet, as this chapter shows, most of these claims turn out to be hard to swallow.

I start this chapter with some basic principles of good nutrition. Although nutritionists are discovering new things about good nutrition all the time, these fundamentals always ring true. One thing you won't find in this chapter is a specific diet or menu plan to follow. Instead, I explain how to personalize and refine the basics so that they make sense for you. I give you some facts, suggestions, and guidelines. Your job is to take this information and make it your own. I also provide a list of the vitamins and minerals your body needs and tell you how much of each to take and where you can find them. Finally, I fill you in on nutritional bars, fast food, and junk food and what they do to and for you. Not sure what to eat to maximize your walking program? Read on.

Fueling Your Body with the Basics

Three fuels — carbohydrates, proteins, and fats — are the body's only sources of calories. No matter what the folks selling food supplements say, these are the only fuels your body can use to produce energy. You need *all three* of these nutrients in your diet to ensure that you get proper nutrition — even fat.

Carbohydrates

Starchy foods, such as pasta, cereal, and rice, are good sources of carbohydrates. Carbohydrates (or *carbs,* as we athletes like to call them) are the nutrient most readily converted into *glycogen,* the elementary fuel your body uses. Carbohydrates are the most efficient form of energy your body has to work with because carbs break down quickly and readily into usable energy. Regardless of what you may read in many popular diet books, carbohydrates should be the mainstay of your diet.

Fifty to seventy percent of your daily calorie intake should come in the form of carbohydrates (more about these percentages in "Playing the Numbers Game," later in this chapter).

Although carbohydrates should be the staple of any healthy diet, be careful about the type of carbs you eat. There are two kinds of carbohydrates: complex carbs (starchy, bready, grainy foods, plus vegetables and legumes) and simple carbs (candy, cake, doughnuts — anything containing large amounts of processed sugar).

Complex carbs are loaded with nutrition. Your body absorbs them slowly, so they provide a steady supply of energy. Simple carbs, on the other hand, are filled with empty, useless calories and are often found in foods that are also high in fat. These carbs are absorbed quickly and affect your energy level like a roller coaster: a quick climb, followed by an equally quick plunge. That's why you feel so low in energy half an hour or so after eating a candy bar or a piece of cake. Fruits and vegetables are a combination of complex and simple carbs; they're healthy because they contain lots of vitamins, minerals, fiber, and water.

Protein

Good sources of protein include meat, poultry, fish, dairy products, soy, legumes, and nuts. Your body uses protein as a backup fuel supply when carbohydrates and fats aren't available.

Proteins are made up of combinations of smaller building blocks called amino acids. Your body needs 22 amino acids to function properly. Nine are called *essential amino acids* because you absolutely must get them from food; the other 13 are called *nonessential* because your body can produce them on its own. If you lack even one essential amino acid, your body starts breaking down muscle tissue to harvest the missing amino acid it needs.

Vegetarians have to be careful because plants contain incomplete proteins, which means that you can't get all your essential amino acids from one source. All the essential amino acids must be present in your meal at one time in order for the body to recombine them into a complete protein. For this reason it is important for vegetarians to combine foods that contain complementary amino acids. Examples of such combinations include rice and beans, peanut butter and whole grain bread, and pasta and vegetables. This type of combination provides the proper mix of amino acids to fulfill protein needs. Vegetarians who include dairy products with their meals are getting all essential amino acids.

Contrary to popular belief, eating excess protein does not help you build muscle and make you stronger. Although muscle tissue is made up primarily of protein, the building block for muscles is energy — not dietary protein. So, to build muscle, eat carbohydrates, which produce a greater deal of energy.

The same holds true for the opposite myth: Eating a lot of protein helps make you thinner. Calories are the key to weight loss, not the type of food those calories come from. If you eat more calories than you burn off — regardless of whether the calories are from steak, corn, or carrot cake — you gain weight.

Only 15 to 30 percent of your caloric intake should come from protein — far less than many popular diet books would have you believe. Actually, protein deficiency is pretty rare in the modern world. If anything, the average person eats *two times the* protein needed. Three modest servings, each about the size of a deck of cards, more than likely cover your protein needs — and then some.

Fat

In spite of their flabby reputation, fats are just as indispensable to your diet as carbs and proteins. Fats provide certain nutrients that are tough to get from any other source. Eating a moderate amount of dietary fat provides energy and helps make you feel full and satisfied. However, most of us don't have to search for ways to add fat to our diets. Most people eat too much fat.

Fat-free and nonfat fats

The term *fat-free* does not mean *calorie-free!* Many fat-free products contain far more calories and sugar than their higher-in-fat counterparts. Plus, they often don't taste as good as the real thing, so you wind up eating more to feel satisfied. Fat-free goodies have never been proved effective for fighting that battle of the bulge. You have to watch how many total calories — not just how many fat calories — you consume.

Some lowfat items do have a place in your diet. In particular, try to eat lowfat dairy products, like lowfat yogurt and skim milk. Other foods earn the lowfat label because they naturally don't contain large amounts of fat. This is a pretty broad category, including everything from pretzels to fruit.

A new twist on fat-free began appearing on your supermarket shelves in 1996. Olestra, the first fake fat, received approval by the Food and Drug Administration (FDA) for human consumption. To date, Frito-Lay's WOW chips are the highest-profile olestra product.

Why are some health advocates up in arms about olestra? Unlike the myriad of other lowfat products, olestra is a real fat — with one notable exception. Whereas the typical natural fat is loaded with 9 calories a gram, olestra is designed to pass right through your body without being digested. An ounce of potato chips fried in olestra has no fat and just 70 calories, compared to 10 grams of fat and 150 calories in conventional chips.

Here's the reason some experts warn against eating large amounts of olestra: When olestra passes through your body, it takes certain nutrients right along with it. Some of these nutrients are thought to protect against cancer. Overconsumption of olestra may also cause cramping and diarrhea, although recent studies have diminished worries about serious gastrointestinal distress.

During an Oprah Winfrey show, an olestra advocate claimed food that is high in fiber also flushes a certain amount of healthful nutrients from the body. Hmmm. While I don't think it will kill you to have an occasional bag of WOW chips, I think it's a bit of a stretch trying to equate fiber with olestra products. My advice: Don't use olestra as an excuse to eat a lot of empty calories and junk food. Eat olestra-based products in moderation, as an occasional treat, until more is known about its long-term effects on the body. The same goes for any food that contains artificial ingredients.

Your fat intake should be 15 to 30 percent of your diet. The average person eats a diet that's closer to 40 percent fat. Too much fat clogs your arteries and is linked to heart disease and numerous types of cancer. The moral of the story here is that you *should* include fat in your diet, but do so with control and some limitations.

Here's the skinny on the three different types of fat in your diet:

> ✔ **Saturated fats:** These fats have all their chemical bonds fully stuffed with hydrogen ions (hence the name *saturated*). They're the true villains that muck up our diets by preventing the liver from filtering out LDL (low-density lipoprotein) cholesterol (otherwise known as "bad"

cholesterol) from the blood. This raises both total cholesterol levels and levels of LDL cholesterol. Saturated fats are easy to recognize because they're solid at room temperature; examples include the fat in your steaks and burgers, butter, cheese, and mayonnaise.

✔ **Monounsaturated fats:** Monounsaturates, such as olive, canola, and peanut oils, seem to be the most effective when substituted for saturated fats because they lower your bad cholesterol without affecting your good cholesterol.

✔ **Polyunsaturated fats:** These fats, including sunflower, corn, soy, and canola oils, do a good job of reducing bad cholesterol levels, but they lower levels of "good" cholesterol (HDL, or high-density lipoprotein), too.

Playing the Numbers Game

Early in this chapter, I give you pretty broad ranges for the amount of each basic nutrient that you should include in your diet: 50 to 70 percent for carbohydrates; 15 to 30 percent for proteins; and 10 to 30 percent for fats. Each person is unique. Whereas one person may lose weight and avoid health problems with a diet that averages 30 percent fat, another person may have to cut fat to around 15 percent to achieve her goals.

Experiment with your diet and see what works best for you. Keep a food diary and analyze it by using a nutrition and calorie book or a nutrition analysis software program. Better yet, take your food diary to a registered dietician and have it professionally critiqued. See how you respond to different percentages of each nutrient in terms of weight loss and energy level. I use the following guidelines to create a unique diet plan for each client:

✔ **Exercise:** The more exercise you do, the more carbs you should include in your diet. If you're a casual, 30-minute, 3-times-a-week walker, you can probably do well on a diet that contains 50 to 60 percent carbohydrates. If you race walk 50 miles a week, you will probably perform better if your diet is closer to 65 to 70 percent carbs.

✔ **Health history:** If you have a history of heart disease, colon cancer, or breast cancer, I recommend keeping your fat intake at the lower end of the spectrum. Ditto if these conditions run in your family. Research shows that a high-fat diet, especially a diet high in saturated fats, may increase your risk of developing these diseases.

✔ **Satiety** (pronounced sah-TIE-a-tee): Satiety is a measure of how full and satisfied you feel after you eat. Some people feel better and eat fewer calories only if their diet runs on the high side of acceptable levels for fat. You will have to manipulate percentages of each nutrient to see how low in fat you can go yet still feel satisfied. But do try to stay within the acceptable ranges for all three basic nutrients.

✔ **Energy level and moods:** Different people react differently to different diets. I work with one woman who feels grouchy unless she has a protein fix in the middle of the afternoon. Other people say they experience a "food hangover" when they overdose on high-carb foods like pasta and bread. Again, keeping a food diary and including a few words on your mood and energy level at various times in the day can help you determine your feel-good foods and your feel-bad foods.

✔ **The foods you eat:** There are many ways to arrive at acceptable nutrient percentages. For instance, if you eat 60 percent carbs, it is probably not wise to achieve this percentage by eating pastas and breads alone. You must eat fruits and vegetables as well. Not all your protein should come from red meat, and not all your fats should be consumed in the form of cake and pie.

Taking a Look at the Food Pyramid

The Food Guide Pyramid (see Figure 4-1), issued by the Food and Drug Administration in 1992, can help you structure your eating. It provides a crystal clear picture of the types and quantities of foods you should eat. And recently it has been updated to make it even more clear and understandable.

The lion's share of your calories should come from the foods at the bottom of the pyramid: grains, cereals, rice, pasta, fruits, and vegetables — those are your carbs. Meat, poultry, fish, eggs, and dairy products fall in the center — those are your proteins. Fats, oils, and sweets are at the very top, under the heading of "use sparingly" — those are your fats. So, you see, the pyramid is really just another way of looking at those percentage recommendations.

To make sure that you don't go overboard on calories, pay attention to what counts as a serving. One serving of meat may mean half a cow to you; however, the federal government's idea of a meat serving, 3 ounces, is about the size of a deck of cards. Here's a rundown of some serving sizes of common foods as defined by the Food Pyramid. You may want to purchase a small, inexpensive kitchen scale to weigh your serving sizes until you learn to eyeball the correct amounts.

✔ **Meat, poultry, fish, dry beans, eggs, nuts:** One serving equals 2 to 3 ounces of lean cooked meat, fish, or poultry; 1 egg; ½ cup cooked beans; or 2 tablespoons seeds and nuts.

✔ **Milk, yogurt, cheese:** One serving equals 1 cup of milk, enough to fill your cereal bowl in the morning; 1 cup of yogurt; or 1½ ounces of cheese, which is about a slice and a half of sliced cheese. (Choose the lowfat varieties.)

✔ **Fruits:** One serving equals one medium apple, banana, or orange; ½ cup of chopped fruit or berries; or ¾ cup of fruit juice. Fresh fruits are usually preferable to frozen, canned, dried, or juiced. However, fresh fruits are not always better than frozen — it depends on how old the "fresh" fruit is. Freezing may do a better job of preserving nutrients.

✔ **Vegetables:** One serving equals 1 cup of raw leafy vegetables; ½ cup of other vegetables such as green beans or carrots, chopped; or ¾ cup vegetable juice.

✔ **Bread, cereal, rice, pasta:** One serving equals 1 slice of bread; 1 ounce of ready-to-eat cereal; or ½ cup of cooked cereal, rice, or pasta.

✔ **Sweets and other high fat foods:** Just keep them to a minimum!

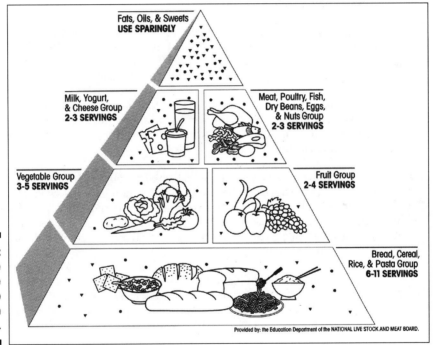

Figure 4-1:
Use the Food Guide Pyramid to help plan your meals.

Fats, Oils, & Sweets
USE SPARINGLY

Milk, Yogurt, & Cheese Group
2-3 SERVINGS

Meat, Poultry, Fish, Dry Beans, Eggs, & Nuts Group
2-3 SERVINGS

Vegetable Group
3-5 SERVINGS

Fruit Group
2-4 SERVINGS

Bread, Cereal, Rice, & Pasta Group
6-11 SERVINGS

Provided by: the Education Department of the NATIONAL LIVE STOCK AND MEAT BOARD.

Keeping Other Nutritional Factors in Mind

If it were just a simple matter of keeping track of your carbs, proteins, and fats, nutrition wouldn't be that complicated. But you need to pay attention to other nutritional considerations also. These other substances don't provide calories per se, but they may impact your health and well-being.

Cholesterol

Animals produce cholesterol in their livers, hence animal fat is the main source of dietary cholesterol. Cholesterol, although it's a form of fat, doesn't contribute extra calories. But it may affect your heart's health in a big, negative way by clogging your arteries, eventually leading to heart disease.

The total fat in your diet, especially saturated fat, can affect your cholesterol levels most dramatically. To lower your blood cholesterol, you need to reduce your fat intake. Talk to your doctor and registered dietician to determine what's right for you.

There are two main types of cholesterol: LDL and HDL. LDL, also known as the "bad" cholesterol, is the substance that clings to the walls of your arteries, blocking them, and forcing your heart to work harder to pump blood through your blood vessels. HDL, the so-called "good" cholesterol, scrubs your artery walls clean, so blood has easy passage and your heart doesn't have to work as hard.

A total cholesterol reading counts both good and bad cholesterol. Any total cholesterol reading of 240 or below is generally considered in the healthy range and puts you at lower risk for heart disease and cancer. It is important to pay attention to your cholesterol ratio. You want your total cholesterol divided by your good cholesterol (HDL) to achieve a ratio of 5:1 or lower. For example, if your total cholesterol is 200 and your HDLs are 66, you divide 200 by 66 for a ratio of about 3:1. Although your total cholesterol number is up at the upper end of the acceptable range, a high level of HDLs balances it out.

Fiber

Fiber refers to the indigestible parts of a plant that help cleanse your digestive system. Most scientific studies have found that eating a diet high in fiber can reduce the risk of colon cancer as well as other types of cancer and health problems. However, the largest study to date did not find a lowered risk of colon cancer.

Fiber comes in two types: insoluble and soluble. Insoluble fiber absorbs water, thereby increasing bulk in your digestive system. This keeps things moving along through your intestines. Soluble fiber dissolves in water, so you fill up more quickly, possibly making weight control easier. Fiber may help lower total cholesterol and blood pressure, too. Whole grains, beans, fruits, and vegetables are good sources of insoluble fiber; whole oats and oat bran are the best sources of soluble fiber.

Most expert organizations agree that you need 20 to 35 grams of fiber daily. A good way to increase your fiber intake is to eat foods as close to their natural state as you can. Carrots, for example, are a pretty good source of fiber. But there's a big difference between raw carrots and carrot cake! Five half-cup servings a day of fresh fruits and vegetables plus three or four servings of whole grain cereal or bread easily meet your fiber requirements.

Don't try to make sudden increases in your fiber intake, especially if you don't eat much fiber right now. Increasing fiber intake too quickly can be a big shock to your system, resulting in gassiness, stomach cramps, and diarrhea. Introduce fiber into your diet slowly. Add an additional gram or two per day until you reach the recommended amount.

Vitamins and minerals

Vitamins come from living sources, such as animals and vegetables. Minerals come from inorganic, or dead, sources that were once part of a large rock or glacier, perhaps the earth's crust. Both are considered *micronutrients* because your body uses them in such small amounts.

Neither vitamins nor minerals give you energy like fats, carbs, or proteins do, but your body needs them in order to perform all the chemical reactions it should. That may not seem like a very big deal until you consider those chemical reactions are responsible for everything from proper breathing to shiny hair.

To keep your body humming along like a well-oiled machine, you need more than 40 essential vitamins and minerals. Although Mother Nature has done a pretty good job packaging these micronutrients in the most advantageous combinations and doses, it is very difficult to achieve the correct balance of vitamins and minerals, especially if you exercise on a regular basis, have a lot of stress in your life, or don't always make the best food choices. That covers just about all of us. For this reason, taking a daily vitamin and mineral supplement is probably a good idea.

A supplement can ensure that you meet your minimum daily requirement for most, if not all, of the essential micronutrients. But don't get any ideas about a little vitamin pill taking the place of a healthy diet. And don't expect a cure for baldness lurking beneath that ball of cotton under the cap either.

Other vitamin and mineral pitfalls to avoid: megadosing and overspending. Because most vitamins are water soluble, that means your body flushes them out of your system instead of storing them. So taking way more than the recommended daily allowance (RDA) only serves to give you very expensive urine! Don't be surprised if your urine turns strange shades of orange, gold, or yellow if you swallow vitamins by the handful. I speak from experience.

Taking large doses of fat-soluble vitamins, primarily A, D and K, can cause serious health problems. Instead of dumping excess amounts, your body stockpiles fat-soluble vitamins in your organs until you're ready to use them. If you overdose on supplements containing fat-soluble vitamins and don't use them quickly enough, they can have serious health side effects, such as increased risk of cancer.

As for overspending, your body doesn't know the difference between a ten-dollar vitamin pill and a ten-cent vitamin pill. I personally can't take adult vitamins because they give me a stomachache even when I take them with food. I pop two Flintstones chewables every morning, and they give me 100 percent of my RDA for all essential vitamins and minerals. A self-proclaimed nutrition expert once gave me flak about this, but I hold that vitamins are vitamins — everything else contained in the pills you buy is filler. So get the best bargain on vitamin and mineral supplements you can; just make sure to check expiration dates because pills do tend to lose potency over time.

Check out Tables 4-1 and 4-2 for information on the vitamins and minerals you need, what they do for your body, how much you should take, and where you can find them.

Table 4-1	Vitamins: What They Do, Where You Can Get Them, and How Much to Take		
Vitamin	*Information about Function and Effects of Deficiency*	*Sources*	*Recommended Daily Allowance (RDA)*
Thiamin (B1)	Without it, you don't burn carbohydrates. It also plays a special role in keeping your heart, nerves, and brain functioning properly.	Lean meats, organ meats, green peas, legumes, whole grains.	Males 15-50: 1.5 mg; Males over 50: 1.2 mg; Females 15-50: 1.1 mg; Females over 50: 1.0 mg
Riboflavin (B2)	Lack of B2 can lead to dry, scaly skin and trouble seeing in bright lights.	Organ meats, dairy products, lean meats, chicken, dark green vegetables, eggs, whole grains, legumes.	Males 15-50: 1.7 mg; Males over 50: 1.4 mg; Females 15-50: 1.3 mg; Females over 50: 1.2 mg

Vitamin	Information about Function and Effects of Deficiency	Sources	Recommended Daily Allowance (RDA)
Niacin (B3)	Keeps LDL cholesterol under control and plays a role in processing carbohydrates. Don't overdose on it though; this can lead to liver damage.	Lean meats, fish, poultry, nuts, legumes, dark green vegetables, whole grains, eggs.	Males 15-50: 19 mg; Males over 50: 15 mg; Females 15-50: 15 mg; Females over 50: 13 mg
Pyridoxine (B6)	Helps break down proteins and is an ingredient in some essential amino acids. Helps pump up your immune system, too.	Lean meat, liver, fish, nuts, legumes, whole grains, poultry, corn, bananas.	Males: 2 mg; Females: 1.6 mg
Cobalamin (B12)	Lack of B12 can lead to anemia (not enough red blood cells.)	Organ meats, lean meat, egg yolks, dairy products, fish, shellfish, poultry.	2.0 mcg
Folic acid	It may lower some birth defects and some experts now think it may lower the risk of heart disease and some cancers.	Meat, dark green, leafy vegetables, asparagus, lima beans, whole grains, nuts, legumes.	Males: 200 mcg; Females: 180 mcg; Pregnant women or trying to conceive: 400 mcg
Ascorbic acid (C)	No proof yet that vitamin C helps prevents colds, but it still may help boost immunity. It helps build healthy bones, teeth, gums and skin. Smokers use up C rapidly, so they should get an extra dose of it.	Strawberries, citrus fruit, cauliflower, broccoli, cabbage, tomatoes, asparagus, green leafy vegetables.	60 mg
Vitamin A	Eat plenty of vitamin A for healthy skin and sharp eyesight.	Liver, eggs, dairy products, dark green vegetables, apricots, peaches, cantaloupes, carrots, squash.	Males: 1,000 RE; Females: 800 RE

(continued)

Table 4-1 *(continued)*

Vitamin	Information about Function and Effects of Deficiency	Sources	Recommended Daily Allowance (RDA)
Vitamin D	Builds strong bones. Helps the body absorb and use calcium and phosphorous.	Milk, egg yolks, salmon with bones, fortified breakfast cereals, sunlight.	Adults over 25: 200 IU
Vitamin E	Lack of E is rare but can cause problems with the nervous system and low birth-weight-infants.	Plant oils, wheat germ, green leafy vegetables, nuts, whole grains, liver, egg yolks, legumes, most other fruits and vegetables.	Adult males: 10 mg (alphatoco-pherols); Adult females: 8 mg (alphatoco-pherols)
Vitamin K	Helps stave off bone density loss and also helps wounds heal. Essential for normal kidney functioning.	Dark green leafy vegetables, asparagus, spinach, turnip greens.	Males: 80 mcg; Females: 65 mcg

Abbreviations:
mg = milligrams   IU=International Units
mcg=micrograms   RE=retinol equivalents (the unit by which vitamin A is measured)

Table 4-2   Minerals: What They Do, Where You Can Get Them, and How Much to Take

Mineral	Information about Function and Effects of Deficiency	Sources	Recommended Daily Allowance (RDA)
Calcium	Keeps your bones and teeth strong, now and in the future. Helps muscles, blood clotting, and nerve function and may help with blood pressure and colon function.	Dairy products, green leafy vegetables, broccoli, fortified orange juice.	Up to age 24: 1,200 mg; After age 24: 800 mg; Postmenopausal, pregnant, and nursing women have increased need.

Mineral	Information about Function and Effects of Deficiency	Sources	Recommended Daily Allowance (RDA)
Chromium	May help Type 2 diabetics regulate their blood sugar.	Brewers yeast, meat, clams, whole grains, cheeses, nuts, eggs.	None, but for adults, 50 to 200 mcg is considered safe and adequate.
Copper	Helps the body make hemoglobin. Helps produce energy in the cells.	Organ meats, shellfish, whole grains, nuts, legumes, lean meat, fish, fruits.	No RDA, but 1.5 to 3.0 mg per day is considered safe and adequate.
Iodine	Helps regulate your metabolism.	Iodized salt, seafood, seaweed.	15 mcg
Iron	Without it, expect a lack of energy due to anemia. (Women in particular are prone to iron deficiencies.)	Organ meats, red meat, fish, shellfish, poultry, enriched cereals, egg yolks, leafy green vegetables, dried fruits.	Males: 10 mg; Females: 15 mg
Magnesium	Fundamental for numerous functions, including energy production.	Whole grains, nuts, legumes, dark green vegetables, seafood, and chocolate.	Males: 350 mg; Females: 280 mg; Pregnant women: 320 to 340 mg
Phosphorus	Essential for strong bones and teeth and healthy skin. Acts as main regulator of energy metabolism. Most Americans get too much of it from soft drinks and processed foods.	Dairy products, fish, meat, poultry, egg yolks, nuts, legumes, whole grains, soft drinks, processed foods.	Teens and adults through age 24: 1,200 mg; Adults 25 and older: 800 mg
Potassium	Regulates the body's fluid balance. Helps keep blood pressure low.	Lean meat, poultry, fresh fruits and vegetables, dairy products, nuts, legumes.	No RDA, but minimum suggested daily intake for adults is 2,000 mg.

(continued)

Table 4-2 *(continued)*

Mineral	Information about Function and Effects of Deficiency	Sources	Recommended Daily Allowance (RDA)
Selenium	Helps the heart and immune system function properly. May help prevent some forms of cancer.	Organ meats, seafood, lean meats, whole grains, dairy products.	Males: 70 mcg; Females: 55 mcg; Pregnant women: 65 mcg Nursing mothers: 75 mcg
Zinc	Men need zinc for proper sperm production. In women, zinc helps normal develop-ment of the fetus. It helps heal wounds and boosts immunity for both sexes.	Meat, poultry, eggs, oysters, dairy products, whole-grain products.	Males: 15 mgs; Females: 12 mg; Pregnant women: 15 mg; Nursing mothers: 19 mg

Abbreviations:
mg = milligrams   mcg=micrograms

Water

Water cools your body, aids circulation and digestion, and carries the fuel used to power your muscles. You need water as much as you need air. In fact, your body is about 60 percent water, and if you lose as little as 2 percent of your body weight through dehydration, your ability to think and move is seriously impaired.

Alcohol, caffeine, sun, heat, wind, exercise, smoking, and air conditioning are just a few of the things that can sap your body of water. Try to drink at least eight, 8-ounce glasses of water to replenish what you lose normally everyday. When you walk, drink two cups of water for every pound you lose from sweating. Your body can absorb only a small amount of liquid at a time, so replace lost water slowly, over the course of a few hours.

Water also comes from other sources, like milk, juice, sports drinks, seltzer, and even juicy fruits. Drinks that don't fully count, and even hurt, are alcohol and caffeinated drinks like coffee, tea, and cola; all of these have a diuretic, or dehydrating, effect.

Many people drink bottled water nowadays. It may taste better than tap water available in your area. However, some new studies show that people who never drink tap water may be at increased risk for tooth decay and gum disease. Tap water, in most parts of the country, is fluoridated, meaning it is supplemented with fluoride, a substance known to protect teeth and gums. Bottled water is usually purified and does not contain added fluoride.

Caffeine

I am one of those people who can't crawl out of bed in the morning without drinking a cup of coffee. Fortunately, my husband understands that I'm not going anywhere until he brings me one. If you're like me, I don't have to tell you that caffeine is classified as a mild stimulant.

Caffeine causes an increase in heart rate and metabolism, which heightens your mental sharpness or, for the more caffeine-sensitive, induces over-the-top jitters. (I can't drink more than my one morning cup without feeling shaky and hyper.) Caffeine reaches the peak of its stimulating powers about 30 minutes after you've had that cup of coffee or tea. It takes your body 4 to 6 hours to metabolize half of your intake. By the way, it takes about 10 hours for caffeine's effects to subside in women who use oral contraceptives. For smokers, it takes about 3 hours.

Most nutritional experts think that caffeine in moderation doesn't do you any harm, but that over-indulging may have a negative impact on your health. Just what overdoing it means depends on your age, health, weight, and caffeine-sensitivity, among other things. Most people are probably okay if they hold their caffeine intake to the equivalent of one to two cups of coffee (150 milligrams) a day. Some studies actually show some possible health benefits to drinking caffeine. A recent study suggested that drinking one to two cups of coffee a day may offer some immunity to gallbladder troubles.

The downside to caffeine: It can leave you feeling agitated and nervous. It can disrupt your ability to concentrate. It can cause diarrhea, dehydration, and irritation. Caffeine can also inhibit your ability to absorb certain nutrients, like thiamin, calcium, and iron. Long-term heavy caffeine use has possible links to breast cancer, colon cancer, and osteoporosis.

Understanding Why Diets Don't Work

Energy from food is measured in calories. Your *basal metabolic rate* (BMR) is the number of calories you need each day to perform basic bodily functions. For an average-size American woman, this number is around 1,000 calories; for the average-size American man, around 1,400. BMR takes into account only the energy your body needs for fundamental functions like breathing, blood circulation, and digestion. It *does not* take into account any movement or exercise you do. Everyday movement generally raises an average person's caloric needs to around 1,600 and 2,000 for women and men, respectively. We walkers burn off even more calories a day through exercise.

Scientists are beginning to believe that your BMR has a *set point,* a certain weight that your body tends to weigh even if you overindulge or make moderate calorie cutbacks. This may be why some people seem to lose weight so easily and others have a harder time trimming off unwanted pounds. However, they also believe that you can exert some influence over your set point. Exercise definitely speeds up your metabolism, especially if you do enough of it to add muscle and drop body fat; some scientists theorize that for each pound of muscle you pack onto your frame, your BMR increases by 50 calories.

One thing does seem clear: The starvation and deprivation method is not the way to rev up your BMR. In fact, it probably slows it down, at least temporarily. When you drastically reduce your caloric intake, your metabolism puts on the brakes. Though you may have initial success with low-calorie diets, the needle on the bathroom scale suddenly stops creeping downward and then stubbornly remains in the same place day after day. When you inevitably quit dieting (as more than 95 percent of people do), your body bounces back to its usual set point. You're no thinner. And you probably feel like a failure because you couldn't lose weight.

This temporary metabolic slowdown is the main reason diets don't work. Just like a car with a nearly empty gas tank, there's too little fuel to run your organic engines properly. You feel hungry all the time and probably lack energy. (That's also why you often feel cold when you're dieting.)

Steer clear of any eating strategy that involves severe restriction or requires you to follow an elaborate set of rules: It's a recipe for disaster. You will fail and feel hungry and miserable the whole time you're dieting. This doesn't mean you shouldn't make an attempt to clean up your eating act. If you eat a giant bowl of pasta every night, as my client Lynn did, you will gain weight. Does that mean that the pasta itself is the culprit and you should banish it from your table altogether? Absolutely not. Limiting portion sizes enables you to enjoy pasta, daily if you like, yet not go overboard on carbohydrates and calories.

Two popular diets have people in my gyms buzzing: The Zone and Sugar Busters. The Zone makes the claim that carbohydrates make you fat, so therefore, you should eat a high-protein diet; Sugar Busters claims that eating sugar is responsible for everything from your excess weight to the national deficit. Of course you can't consume mountains of carbs or scarf down sugary treats by the pound. But that doesn't mean these wacky diets can fix your weight problem, increase your energy level, or make all your health troubles disappear.

People often have initial success on these two diet plans — as well as nearly every other fad diet — because they both restrict calories. You lose weight because you eat less, not because you have unlocked some magical secret that helps melt away body fat.

Outlining Special Eating Strategies for Walkers

If you're really interested in losing weight, walking is a great way to start. The following list of eating strategies can help you as well. Walkers should follow the same fundamental nutritional rules as everyone else, and pay attention to these special tips:

 ✔ **Eat before you walk.** Forget what your mother told you. You need to eat before you exercise. Eat a small, high-carb meal half an hour to an hour before you head out the door so that your blood sugar is in full swing during your walk. You'll have more energy and feel better than if you skipped the snack. The best pre-workout choices are starchy, complex carbohydrates like bagels, whole grain bread, and rice. Experiment with different foods. If you tossed back a handful of crackers and they made you feel crampy during your walk, try a piece of raisin toast next time out.

 You don't have to eat a ton, just enough to give you that extra energy boost. Overdoing portion size works against you. Also, this is one time you may want to avoid some otherwise healthy foods. Eat a high-fiber snack or an acidic piece of fruit and you may find yourself doubled over 20 minutes into your walk.

 ✔ **Eat after you walk.** You need to replenish your glycogen stores after a good workout, so make sure that you eat a small snack after your walk. Again, reach for those carbs. At this point, juicy fruits are a good choice because they replace carbs, water, and electrolytes. Even if you aren't hungry — exercise can dull the appetite — grab a piece of fruit and take a few bites. You can always eat a heartier meal later on.

 ✔ **Eat while you walk.** As crazy as this sounds, you may need to eat at some point during a walk. Of course, you shouldn't be wolfing down a turkey sandwich to fuel a 20-minute jaunt around the neighborhood. But if you're doing a 4-hour hike or an all-day walkathon, it's wise to bring a snack along. Hikers should pack snacks that are high in protein and fat to replace all the calories they burn off. Gorp is a standard hiking snack; the name is shorthand for Good Old Raisins and Peanuts. Long-distance walkers should keep a simple carb handy. Candy, yes *candy,* is a good mid-to-end race choice because it gives you a quick shot of energy when you need it most.

 ✔ **Drink lots of water.** It is essential to drink before, during, and after your walk. Carry water with you and take a sip every few minutes, even if you don't feel thirsty. By the time you do feel that thirst, you're already partially dehydrated. When the weather is extremely hot and humid or you're walking for more than an hour, consider sipping a sports drink like Gatorade or Powerade. The electrolyte and carbs they contain help replenish what you lose from sweat.

Dissecting sports nutrition bars

I once went to a fitness trade show and was stunned to see an entire exhibit hall the size of a warehouse devoted to sports nutrition bars. I opened my plastic bag and yelled, "Trick or treat" every time someone tossed another sample in my bag. When I got home and spread them out on my desk, I was even more stunned to find that I had collected over 40 different brands of these things.

Examining the labels of these bars was a true education for me. One claimed to be formulated to meet the special needs of women. Another claimed to be formulated to meet the special needs of tennis players. Yet another claimed to mimic the nutritional content of mother's milk.

I opened one up and took a bite, and you know, it was pretty good. In fact, too good. It was coated with a thick layer of chocolate and tasted just like a candy bar. Of course, others weren't so good; some had the taste and texture of wet plywood coated with rubber cement.

Tasty or not, most of the nutritional bars I have sampled pack just as much sugar and as many calories as any candy bar you find at your local candy counter. One particularly tasty bar claimed to be packed with muscle-building protein, but it also contained 240 calories and 10 grams of fat, and listed the main ingredient as dextrose, a form of processed sugar. By comparison, a Milky Way candy bar of approximately the same weight contains 250 calories, 9.1 of them from fat. It contains less sugar and nearly as much protein as this so-called nutritional supplement bar.

I don't object to treating yourself to an occasional nutrition bar as a snack or when you don't have time for a meal. But don't kid yourself. Most of them are nothing more than high-priced candy bars with a vitamin coating and a little extra protein thrown in. If you take a daily multivitamin and eat well, you don't need to eat these pseudo candy bars.

✔ **Manipulate your carbs.** Walkers who go at a moderate pace for under 30 minutes a workout can probably stay on the low end of the carbohydrate range in their diet; 50 to 60 percent of their calories should come from carbs. Walkers who put in more time and mileage may need to up their carb intake for optimal performance. Once again, experiment here. Keep a food diary and analyze it regularly so that you can pinpoint the balance of carbs, fat, and protein that makes you feel best. Your carb intake may change as your workouts change.

✔ **Don't use walking as an excuse to pig out.** Yes, you burn an average of 100 calories a mile as you walk, but that doesn't give you a license to go hog wild. Your walking program is an important part of a weight-loss program, but it can't perform miracles. If you eat more than you burn off, you're gonna gain weight.

Avoiding Fast Food and Junk Food

Food that you order by speaking into the mouth of a clown or that comes in glow-in-the-dark colors are, unfortunately, a growing part of the average person's diet. Typically, fast foods and junk foods are laden with extra fat, salt, and calories but light on nutritional value. And, although it's okay to splurge on an occasional fast-food meal or stroll down the candy aisle of the supermarket, here are a few rules to help you avoid making a disaster of your diet.

Fast food

The best rule to keep in mind when you pull up to the drive-through to place your order is to keep it simple. Avoid specialty sandwiches with globs of special sauce, and stick to pared-down, basic sandwiches or junior versions. Lose the words "cheese" and "double" from your order. Chicken and fish may seem like healthy alternatives, but if they're fried or batter-dipped, they rival specialty burgers in terms of fat and calories. That's true for anything that comes in chunk or nugget form as well.

Many fast-food joints now offer lowfat burger options, although the McDonald's McLean burger proved to be a dud with consumers. Better-tasting, lowfat options include a barbecued chicken sandwich or a plain salad. Just go easy on the extras they put in salads, including processed meats, cheese, hard-boiled eggs, and creamy dressings.

For fast-food breakfasts, go with pancakes or an English muffin (hold the butter if you can stand it), orange juice, and lowfat milk. As for lunch, if you can, resist the 200 plus calories and 50 percent fat of a regular order of French fries. Go for the hot apple pie or chocolate shake instead. Though these two items offer nearly the same number of calories as the fries, more than half of their calories are from carbs and less than 30 percent come from fat.

The best type of fast food can be found at pizza and Mexican chains. A slice of pizza is around 70 percent carbs and 20 percent fat (calories vary by slice size, of course). Likewise for a bean burrito, unadorned taco, or an order of rice and beans with a sprinkle of cheese. You do have to be careful, though. Taco Bell has one sandwich that weighs in at over 2,000 calories and 60 percent fat.

Junk food

Munchies that hit you while you're studying, right after you put the baby to sleep, or when you're working late at the office can be overpowering. You want something, and it's got to be crunchy, smooth and creamy, or sweet.

If you crave crunchy, you may be tempted to reach for a bag of potato chips. Unfortunately, a measly 2-ounce bag of potato chips offers 306 calories, 58 percent of them from fat. You can blow a whole day's virtues in one swift handful. Nuts and seeds, though "natural," are even worse. It runs you 320 calories for two ounces of peanuts, and 77 percent of those calories are from fat, even more for the same amount of cashews or macadamia nuts.

Your safest crunchy munchie is a bag of pretzels. Unlike chips and nuts, they're high in carbs, relatively low in calories, and only 6 percent fat. Popcorn can be a good choice too, but be careful here. Air-popped without butter and salt offers just 20 lowfat calories per cup. The same amount of microwave or oil-popped popcorn may deliver as many as 110 calories and 8 grams of fat. Movie theater popcorn is one of the worst choices you can make. A large popcorn can contain more than a thousand calories and as much saturated fat as you get from five fast-food specialty burgers — and that's before you add the butter flavoring.

One of my clients told me that when he craves something crunchy, he eats raw new potatoes; those are the small, hard red variety of potato. This man swears by them, but I don't know. . . I don't think that would cut it for me. Perhaps you have your own healthy crunchy snack?

For smooth and creamy cravings, a cup of fruit-flavored, lowfat frozen yogurt is the safest selection (around 225 calories, 10 percent fat). However, the nutrition information displayed in a yogurt shop or on a yogurt container usually applies to vanilla flavor and to portion sizes that are much smaller than what is typically served. Other flavors, especially those with nuts or other add-ins, contain more fat and calories. Frozen yogurt vendors can sometimes be misleading about fat, calorie, and sugar content and the serving sizes of their products. Be sure to read labels and decipher serving sizes carefully.

I don't usually recommend fat-free products, but many of the fat-free ice creams actually taste pretty good; they are significantly lower in fat and calories than regular ice cream but are still delicious and filling enough to satisfy a yearning for ice cream. Edy's, Dreyer's and Turkey Hill make a fat-free, sugar-free ice cream that is surprisingly good. Just make sure that you stick to a serving size. Don't eat the whole pint at one sitting.

When your sweet tooth starts sending you signals, fig bars are your wisest cookie option (two have 110 calories, 17 percent fat). Angel food cake is also a good choice, weighing in at 140 calories per heavenly slice. My Mom loves Gummy Bears; she can eat just a few, and they satisfy her. Although you can eat the lowfat and no-fat versions of your favorite sweet treats, read the labels carefully. Sometimes they're not the fat and calorie bargain you think they are. Also, because they don't taste as good as the real deal, you tend to eat more of them.

Chapter 5

Walking Logistics

. . . .

In This Chapter

▶ Understanding the four levels of walking

▶ Using the FIT formula to structure your walking program

▶ Following safety rules

▶ Venturing out in all sorts of weather

. . . .

*I*n this book, I describe four different levels of walking. In fact, I devote a chapter to each of them (see Chapters 7 through 10). Depending on your goals, you may include all four levels in your program, or you may only include one or two. That's the beauty of walking: It's infinitely adaptable. You can modify and mold a walking program to accommodate your individual fitness level, goals, and abilities.

Besides deciding on a walking level, you also need to consider the structure of your walking program. How hard should you work during a walk? How often should you walk? How long should each walk take you? I answer these and other questions in this chapter. In addition, I offer tips on how to make your walking program safer and more enjoyable.

The Four Levels of Walking

Here is a brief description of the four levels of walking that I refer to throughout this book. The walking level you choose relates to much of the information contained in this chapter and is the basis for your entire workout plan. You can find out more about each level of walking in detail by reading the corresponding chapters that follow in Part II of the book.

Level 1 — Lifestyle walking

Lifestyle walking is the type of casual walking you do when you stroll through the park or the mall. It's a relatively low-intensity activity, but that doesn't mean it isn't good for you. Lifestyle walking is a good entry-level fitness activity and a sensible starting point for your walking program if you haven't exercised in a while. Most lifestyle walkers walk an average of 2.5 to 3.5 miles per hour, meaning that you cover one mile every 17 to 24 minutes. Because lifestyle walking is the most straightforward of all walking techniques, it's perfect for beginners who want to help build stamina and muscular strength. Focus on this level if your goal is long-term health and an improved quality of life. I recommend lifestyle walking as a part of every walker's program because a truly successful health and fitness plan must include an increase in overall movement and daily activity.

Level 2 — Fitness walking

Walkers exercising on the treadmill at the gym or high-stepping through the neighborhood are engaged in fitness walking. Fitness walking is a perfect low-impact way to get fit and stay fit. It's an excellent weight loss activity with little risk of injury. You can use it as your main fitness activity if your goals are moderate weight loss, improved health, increased energy, and longevity. Fitness walkers typically move along at a brisk pace of 3.5 to 4.3 miles an hour, covering a mile in a respectable 14 to 17 minutes. Fitness walking utilizes the hips, buttocks, lower back, abdominals, and upper body muscles.

Level 3 — High-energy walking

This form of walking is a great calorie burner and muscle shaper. It's a takeoff on the sport of race walking. High-energy walkers zip along at a lightning-fast pace of 4.4 to 6.0 miles an hour, covering a mile in a blazing 10 to 13.6 minutes. You should include at least some high-energy walking in your program if your goals are increased muscle tone and improved athletic performance, and if you're looking for a calorie burn similar to running but without the high risk of injury. Most walkers use high-energy walking as a hard-day aerobic activity rather than their mainstay workout, although some walkers get addicted to it and use it as their primary cardio workout.

Level 4 — Walk-Run

Walk-run is the perfect hybrid activity for walkers who have the need for speed but don't want to greatly pump up their risk of injury. Walk-run involves alternating running intervals and walking intervals in order to spike up exercise intensity, work more muscles, and burn more calories. Although you never have to run a single step to get in fantastic shape, you may want to try a walk-run workout at least once in a while. It's just another way to get more bang for your fitness buck. If, however, even short jogging stints make your knees ache, stick with pure walking. As I explain in Chapter 10, you can substitute high-energy walking intervals for the running intervals and get a similar workout.

Structuring Your Walking Program with the FIT Formula

Variable is nothing more than a fancy word for an aspect of your walking program that you can adjust. You can play around with three different variables to make your walking and total fitness program harder or easier. I recommend using the FIT variables to structure your walking program: Frequency, Intensity, and Time.

Changing one of these workout variables affects the others. For instance, if you work out harder, you are increasing your intensity and, as a result, may not be able to work out for as long or as often. When you increase the time you spend walking, you may not be able to work out as often or at the same level of effort. The secret to designing a walking routine that works for you is to strike the right balance of all three aspects of the FIT formula.

Before you can begin manipulating each FIT variable, you need to understand what each variable is. Throughout this book I help you take these principles and relate them to all the walking levels. I explain how to juggle them in order to get the perfect balance of the three for a walking and total exercise program that suits your needs, goals, and fitness level.

Frequency

Frequency refers to the number of times you work out per week. The number of your weekly workouts often has a direct impact on how quickly you achieve your goals.

The American College of Sports Medicine, among other respected organizations, recommends that everyone do some sort of activity that exercises the heart at least three times a week. At this minimum level of activity, you can achieve certain health goals, such as increased stamina, lower cholesterol, and protection from heart disease and other forms of chronic illness. However, if your goal is to lose weight or train for an athletic event, you need to walk more often to achieve results.

The type of walking you do may also dictate the number of times that you need to exercise per week. If you're a lifestyle walker, try to walk every day or nearly every day because lifestyle walking is a relatively low-intensity activity. On the other hand, if your primary form of walking is high-energy or walk-run — two activities at the more intense end of the walking scale — take at least one day off a week to prevent injury and workout burnout.

Intensity

When you see a high-energy walker zipping by, notice that she's breathing pretty hard and has a nice sweat going. When a lifestyle walker strolls by, however, he looks comfortable and relaxed. The difference between these two walkers is their workout intensity. The word intensity means how hard you're working.

You can measure intensity in three ways: You can take your heart rate, rate your level of exertion by using a tool called the RPE scale, or take the talk test. Familiarize yourself with all three ways and decide for yourself which way works best for you.

Heart rate

Measuring your heart rate during your workout is the most precise way to track exercise intensity. How fast your heart beats corresponds directly with how hard you're working. Your goal is not to hit an exact heart rate each time you work out but rather an entire range of heart rates. This range is called your *target heart rate zone.*

Your target heart rate zone is the range of heart rates your heart should be beating for a given intensity of exercise. The range is based on your maximum heart rate, or the fastest your heart is able to beat under any circumstances.

If you are taking any medications, get your doctor's advice about what your maximum heart rate and training zone should be. Some medications affect how fast your heart can beat, even if you're working very hard. Also, if you are pregnant or have a medical condition, your doctor may want to dictate how hard you should be working out.

To estimate your maximum heart rate, subtract your age from 220. Next, multiply this number by 0.5 and .95 to come up with your walking target heart rate range. The intensity of effort that you shoot for during a workout is usually within a narrow band of this broad target heart rate zone.

- ✔ When you're lifestyle walking, aim for a target heart rate zone between 50 and 60 percent of your maximum heart rate.
- ✔ When you're fitness walking, aim for a target heart rate range between 60 and 75 percent of your maximum heart rate.

✔ When you high-energy walk, aim for a target heart rate range of 75 to 95 percent of your maximum heart rate.

✔ When you walk-run, aim for a variable target heart rate that spans your entire target range, depending on whether you are running or walking easily to recover from a run.

Without regular monitoring, you may think that you're exercising at a certain intensity, but in fact, you may not be. You may discover that you're not working hard enough, or if you're trying to take it easy, you may be working out harder than you think. In that case, measuring your heart rate lets you know that you need to slow down. This instantaneous precision allows you to more easily fine-tune your workout levels.

You can measure your heart rate, or pulse, at your wrist or the base of your neck. At your wrist, you simply place your index and middle finger lightly on the vein below your thumb. Or you can place your index and middle fingers on the groove at the side of your neck, count the number of beats you feel in 15 seconds, and multiply by 4.

If all this poking, prodding, and math seem too complicated to you, you may want to purchase a heart rate monitor. The best, most accurate heart rate monitors consist of a chest strap and wristwatch. You fasten the strap around you, just below your chest, and the strap transmits your heart rate to the watch via electromagnetic waves. Heart rate monitors have been perfected over the years so that they are now nearly as accurate as the machines that doctors use to measure your heart rate. I like Polar heart rate monitors the best; they are reliable and reasonably priced at around $70 to start.

Take your heart rate after you've been working out for at least 5 minutes. If you exercise for 30 minutes or more, take your heart rate every 15 to 20 minutes or so. You may also find it useful to take your recovery heart rate, which is your heart rate 1 minute after you stop exercising. The faster your heart rate slows down, the better condition you're in.

If you thrive on feedback, tracking the rhythms of your heart can be motivational. As you get fitter, your heart doesn't have to work as hard at a given workload, so monitoring your pulse lets you know whether you're getting in better shape. Monitoring your heart rate also tells you how fast your heart rate recovers at the end of your workout and between hard-driving intervals.

Rating of perceived exertion

Having an overall sense of how hard you think you're working is a good way to measure intensity. The RPE (short for *rating of perceived exertion*) scale (see Table 5-1) helps put a number on your general psychological impressions of intensity by rating it on a scale of 1 to 10.

A 1 on the RPE scale represents a level of activity that is really, really easy. You could do a 1 activity all day without feeling winded, and it's no more effort than sitting in bed, watching TV, and eating popcorn. At the other end of the scale, a 10 represents a maximum level of activity. It's like you've just run all out for the past hour straight uphill and can't possibly take another step. Obviously, you need to strive for a level of activity that falls somewhere in between a 1 and a 10.

- ✔ For lifestyle walking, an RPE of 4 to 6 is ideal.
- ✔ For fitness walking, an RPE of 6 to 8 is ideal.
- ✔ For high-energy walking, an RPE of 8 to 9.5 is ideal.
- ✔ For walk-run, strive for an RPE of anywhere from 4 to 9.5, depending on what phase of the workout you're in.

Table 5-1	RPE Scale
Numerical Rating	*Subjective Rating*
0	Nothing at all
0.5	Very, very weak
1	Very weak
2	Weak
3	Moderate
4	Somewhat strong
5	Strong
6	
7	Very strong
8	
9	
10	Very, very strong

The talk test

The talk test is the simplest way to gauge exercise intensity. By talking aloud as you walk, you can tell how hard you're working. If you can yodel while you're walking, you aren't working hard enough. If you barely breathe — let alone utter a syllable — you're working too hard. Here are some talk test guidelines:

✔ You should be able to carry on a slightly breathy conversation during a lifestyle walk.

✔ You should be able to offer snatches of breathless conversation during a fitness walk.

✔ You should barely be able to speak during the peak of your high-energy walking workouts, although you should be able to throw out a breathless word or two here or there.

✔ Your talk test will vary during your walk-run, depending on whether you are involved in a high-intensity or low-intensity phase.

Time

The last part of the FIT formula is time, or how long your walks last. The length of your workouts is dictated by many factors:

✔ **Frequency:** You may choose to walk more often instead of doing a long workout three or four days a week. Once again, fiddling with the FIT formula so that it works for you is fine, as long as you can actually achieve your goals and derive health benefits from your plan.

✔ **Intensity:** The higher intensity your workouts, the shorter they will be. You can't keep up very high-intensity exercise for long periods of time. On the other hand, if your walks are pretty low-key, you should be able to walk for an hour or more without feeling so tired that you have to stop.

✔ **Schedule:** You may not have an hour every day to walk. If your time is of the essence, then that factor probably dictates the length of your walks. However, you always have the option of splitting your walks up into two or three mini-sessions a day.

✔ **Fitness level:** The fitter you are, the longer you can walk. When you first start out, you may get winded after 20 minutes. After you've been exercising for a while, you may be able to go as long as 45 minutes without getting tired.

✔ **Goals:** Sometimes your goals will determine how much time you spend walking. I have a client who is training for a trekking trip in the Grand Canyon. She walks for several hours a day a couple of times a week in preparation for that trip. Many other clients do a quick 20-minute walk for health purposes before they head off to pump iron or take a yoga class.

Safety First

Everyone — male, female, young, old — must take certain precautions to ensure a safe walk, whether it's in a crowded city, the suburbs, or rural areas. To a certain extent, your lifestyle and your neighborhood dictate your safety concerns. A busy mom may be able to squeeze in a midmorning walk around the neighborhood after the kids have gone to school and before starting her errands. An executive who works long hours may only have time to walk after dinner on the streets near his apartment. Both can and should take certain precautions before heading out the door.

I have a woman friend who walks in Central Park a couple nights a week. Even though several well-publicized cases of rape and assault have occurred on women in this beautiful but somewhat unsafe New York City park in the past few years, she insists on going it alone. When I ask her about it, she asserts that women should be able to walk anywhere, anytime. Otherwise, they let the criminals win, she says. Although I certainly agree with her position in theory, the sad reality is that your workout, though important, isn't worth risking your life over.

Regardless of where you walk, pay careful attention to the following safety tips. They apply to all walkers, all the time.

- ✔ **Walk defensively.** Don't ever challenge a vehicle or assume that drivers, cyclists, skaters, and other pedestrians understand when you have the right of way. Don't ever take it for granted that someone has seen you and will yield, even if you have made eye contact. When in doubt, always err on the side of caution, regardless of wheher you legally have the right of way.

- ✔ **Whenever possible, walk on a bike path or in an area where motorized traffic is not allowed.** However, if you have no such luxury, always walk facing traffic and along the shoulder of the road. The only exception to this rule is blind curves and narrow turns. In those instances, carefully cross to the side of the road that affords you the best view of traffic and cross back to the other side when it is safe to do so.

- ✔ **When you walk alone, let someone know where you're going.** I give my proposed route and the approximate time of my return to someone before I leave. Always carry identification and important medical information with you. Both may be vital if you get hurt are and unable to communicate this information yourself.

- ✔ **Don't walk alone at night, especially in secluded areas.** If you must walk after dark for the sake of convenience, consider joining a walking club or group. Not one in your area? Start your own. This rule applies not only to women. Men who exercise alone at night are just as vulnerable to muggers and thieves.

✔ **If you must walk at night, wear white or brightly colored clothing with some type of reflective material to increase the chance of being seen by oncoming motorists, cyclists, and skaters.** This same advice holds true for foggy weather as well. Whenever you have the option, walk in brightly lit areas.

✔ **If possible, vary your route and the time of day you walk.**

✔ **Leave your personal stereo at home.** Tuning out with some tunes can be relaxing, but it is very dangerous when you're walking. You can't hear oncoming traffic, someone coming up behind you, or any other noises. Studies also show that using personal stereos, especially at high volumes, causes hearing impairment. Save your personal stereo for your gym and other indoor workouts.

Okay. I know that many of you are going to break this rule. If you absolutely, positively must use a personal stereo when you walk, keep the volume low. Scan your environment often and don't zone out so completely that you are totally unaware of your surroundings.

✔ **Be alert when walking past dense brush, wooded areas, doorways, and courtyards.** Avoid them whenever possible. (I realize, of course, that avoiding wooded areas during a hike is impossible.) I strongly suggest that you never hike alone, no matter how familiar you are with a trail.

✔ **Don't wear a lot of jewelry or carry a lot of money when you walk.** A dollar's worth of change allows you to make a phone call in an emergency.

✔ **Some experts advocate carrying mace or some other self-defense device.** Only do so if you are prepared to use it. I used to work with a self-defense expert who advocated carrying a large knife when exercising alone outdoors. He even bought me one as a gift and showed me how to use it. But I never could get comfortable with this idea. I was always afraid that I would lose my nerve if confronted and that an attacker might be able to get the knife away from me. The last thing anyone wants is to give an attacker a weapon to use against him! I put the knife away in a safe place and have never used it. But I do know several walkers who carry some form of self-defense. A good compromise is a police whistle. You can attract attention and possibly scare an attacker away without increasing your chances of injury.

✔ **If you feel vulnerable because of your age, sex, or the area where you walk but you can't find a walking companion, consider the mall (see Chapter 17) or a gym as an alternative.** Most of us love to get out and move around in the great outdoors — but it's no fun when you don't feel relaxed.

Walking in All Kinds of Weather

The ups and downs of the thermometer can greatly affect how you feel during your walk. I know I tend to wilt like an old flower arrangement when I exercise outdoors in hot weather. Ironically, I do most of my workouts indoors during the summer months, while most other people make an effort to get out and exercise in the warm sun. But before the first snowflake touches down, I have my shoes laced up and I'm out the door. If snow makes footing treacherous, I wait for the snowplow and walk behind it.

Braving the elements can be a joy, the sort of satisfaction from being out there doing your thing in spite of the curveballs nature throws at you. I have often gone out for a workout in a raging rainstorm, and even though I've returned home soaked to the skin, I've felt good about my efforts. (Once I even went for a walk with my dog in a hailstorm, but I admit that was just nutty.)

Don't let a little natural adversity keep you from your appointed rounds. Do keep in mind, however, the special considerations each change in the weather brings. If you prepare for them, you can exercise safely and comfortably in just about every circumstance.

Cool tips for walking in hot weather

Of all the types of weather you may run into, hot, humid weather has perhaps the greatest capacity for danger. On a really steamy, hot day, you can overheat and dehydrate very quickly, especially if you're just getting back into shape.

If you heed just one piece of advice about walking in hot weather, make it this: Drink tons of water. Your body can absorb only about half as much water as you sweat off while you're working out, so you need to drink liberally and often. You know that old rule about drinking eight glasses of water a day? When you exercise in the heat, you should probably drink closer to ten. Forget about popping salt tablets though. Most of us get plenty of salt from our diets — even those of us who sweat like pigs.

Always carry a water bottle or some other type of water carrier. Drink as often as you feel thirsty or more often if you can stand it. Continue to drink after your workout, too, even if you aren't thirsty. It will help you stay hydrated. I like to fill my water bottle up halfway with ice cubes and the rest of the way with water or a sports drink so that I always have something refreshing and cool to drink.

JARGON ALERT

Heat humidity index

The *apparent temperature* refers to how hot the combination of heat and humidity make you feel. When heat and humidity combine to reduce the amount of evaporation of sweat from the body, outdoor exercise becomes dangerous, even for those in good shape. Here is the heat humidity index based on the apparent temperature.

■ **Extreme danger**   ■ **Danger**   □ **Extreme caution**   ■ **Caution**

RELATIVE HUMIDITY (PERCENT)

AIR TEMP	0	5	10	15	20	25	30	35	40	45	50	55	60	65	70	75	80	85	90	95	100
140	125																				
135	120	128																			
130	117	122	131																		
125	111	116	123	131	141																
120	107	111	116	123	130	139	148														
115	103	107	111	115	120	127	135	143	151												
110	99	102	105	108	112	117	123	130	137	143	150										
105	95	97	100	102	105	109	113	118	123	129	135	142	149								
100	91	93	95	97	99	101	104	107	110	115	120	126	132	138	144						
95	87	88	90	91	93	94	96	98	101	104	107	110	114	119	124	130	136				
90	83	84	85	86	87	88	90	91	93	95	96	98	100	102	106	109	113	117	122		
85	78	79	80	81	82	83	84	85	86	87	88	89	90	91	93	95	97	99	102	105	108
80	73	74	75	76	77	77	78	79	79	80	81	81	82	83	85	86	86	87	88	89	91
75	69	69	70	71	72	72	73	73	74	74	75	75	76	76	77	77	78	78	79	79	80
70	64	64	65	65	66	66	67	67	68	68	69	69	70	70	70	70	71	71	71	71	72

AIR TEMPERATURE (DEGREES FAHRENHEIT)

Apparent temperature *is how hot the heat-humidity combination makes it feel.*

Source: National Oceanic and Atmospheric Administration

DUMMIES APPROVED

Choose walking clothing made of fabrics such as CoolMax and Supplex that pull moisture away from your body. They allow sweat to evaporate quickly, leaving you feeling cooler and cleaner. Most sporting goods stores and large department stores sell walking and running clothing made from these fabrics. Wear lighter colors because they keep you cooler. I am also a big fan of synthetic mesh because the holes allow moisture to escape, yet they also catch any breeze that happens to blow by. In fact, you'll actually be cooler in a mesh T-shirt than if you go shirtless.

Sunblock is a must to protect your skin from sunburn. Many good sunblocks on the market are formulated especially for exercise and sweating. I buy the no-name brands you can get at almost any drugstore because they're inexpensive and work just as well as the pricey brands. Combine sunscreen with a hat to protect your scalp, and a good pair of sunglasses to protect your eyes.

When the heat is on, give yourself permission to back off on your pace and/or your distance. Hot weather can sap your strength and stamina because your body works so hard to cool itself off. If you overdo it, the three following conditions are potential results:

- ✔ **Heat cramps:** This is a seizing up of one or more of your muscles, often the calves. It's often the first sign of heat-related trouble. If you don't pay attention, cramps are a small symptom of things to come. If you experience heat cramps, stop and get into the shade if possible. Gently massage the affected muscle, carefully stretch out, and apply ice if it's available.

- ✔ **Heat exhaustion:** This malady is characterized by profuse sweating, cold and clammy skin, and a weak and rapid pulse. Your skin may be pale, and you may feel sick and dizzy. In extreme cases, you may lose consciousness. If you experience these symptoms, move into the shade as soon as possible. Lie down and elevate your feet about 12 to 18 inches. Drink plenty of fluids and monitor your pulse. See a doctor as soon as possible for further treatment.

- ✔ **Heatstroke:** This is the most serious of all heat-related injuries. At this point, you stop perspiring, and your skin is very hot and dry to the touch. You are either flushed or, if you are a person of color, ashen. You have a strong, rapid pulse and difficulty breathing. These symptoms call for immediate medical attention. Remove as much clothing as possible without exposing yourself to the sun. Cool down as quickly as possible with any method available — water, a fan, air conditioning, or ice packs. Wrap yourself in cold wet sheets for transportation to the hospital or doctor.

Taking it easy helps prevent these heat-related illnesses. Acclimate yourself to warmer weather for about a week. When the first heat wave of the year hits, back off for a few days and gradually build up to your normal level of walking.

Dressing for a winter wonderland

A few years back, I showed up for a mid-February marathon in upstate New York dressed in a short-sleeved T-shirt and a pair of nylon running shorts. It was a sunny, breezy 50 degrees at the start, but at about mile 15, the clouds started rolling in; by mile 20, we were running through a full-fledged blizzard. Thanks to zero visibility, I missed mile marker 25 and ran 2 miles off course before a volunteer tracked me down and rerouted me in the right direction. I eventually hobbled across the finish line, teeth chattering, legs frozen, with early stages of frostbite on the tips of my ears and fingers.

Such are the perils of running and walking outdoors in the winter. Still, many of us would rather brave a little snow and wind chill than stay cooped up in a stuffy gym or airless basement till the spring thaw. With a few precautions (which *I* clearly didn't follow), a winter walk in the great outdoors need not be such a harrowing experience.

The big secret to walking outdoors in the winter is to wear as little as possible. No, I'm not talking about walking in your underwear. You want to wear as little as you can get by with and still be comfortable after you get moving. Your clothing should cover as much surface area of your body as possible and protect you from the three major elements of winter weather: cold, wind, and precipitation. So, instead of wearing one or two pieces of big, bulky clothing, you're better off wearing three thin layers. Here's what I suggest:

- ✔ For the innermost layer, choose a material made from polypropylene or olefin. Both are better at wicking perspiration away from your skin than natural fibers like cotton or wool, which tend to get damp and clammy with sweat.

- ✔ The second layer serves as an insulator. A loose, lightweight sweater, sweatshirt, or long-sleeved T-shirt traps warm air generated by your body heat but lets you move without restriction; Gore-Tex works well because it breathes, but natural fibers are also good choices.

- ✔ A light, easy-to-open jacket acts as a shield from the wind, rain, and snow. Look for a garment that's both breathable and waterproof — that is, something that allows your sweat to evaporate yet still prevents outside moisture from seeping through. Gore-Tex and other synthetics are your best bet.

- ✔ Shed a layer or open up your jacket zipper as soon as you feel too hot so that body heat can escape and air may circulate freely.

- ✔ Keep your legs fully covered but don't overdo it. When you exercise, a tremendous amount of blood is shunted to the legs, and their metabolism increases dramatically. Thermal underwear and a pair of tights are almost always adequate.

- ✔ Your head and hands are prime frostbite targets, so finish off your outer gear with a hat and mittens (which keep your hands warmer than gloves). Add a face guard or bandanna if it's windy. And just because it's cold out doesn't mean that you can skip the sunblock: You'll burn just as quickly from the combination of wind and sun reflecting off the snow as you will from a day at the beach.

You have struck the right balance of clothing if you feel slightly chilly when you first step outside but are sufficiently toasty after about 10 minutes of exercise.

Obviously, checking the weather report before you head out the door is a good idea. Winter weather can change dramatically in a matter of minutes. If you follow these basic rules, your chance of feeling uncomfortable or — worst case scenario — ending up with hypothermia or frostbite is extremely remote.

Treading carefully on snow and ice

You can't always tell what kind of terrain is underneath snow cover. As a result, if you're not careful to keep your eyes peeled on the road ahead, you may be surprised by a pothole or slick patch of ice. Icy hills are especially dangerous. During a particularly treacherous winter several years ago, the going was so slippery that diehard runners and walkers were crawling up the Brooklyn Bridge's inclined footpath and sliding down the other side.

Lateral stability on snow, slush, and ice presents a real opportunity for injury; you can easily twist an ankle or turn your knee in an attempt to stay upright. High snowdrifts and unplowed streets require an extra effort, too, especially from your buttocks and thigh muscles. Take shorter, quicker strides than normal and hold your arms slightly away from your body to improve your balance. Whenever possible, travel along well-worn paths where the snow cover is minimal and you can see what's coming up.

If footing isn't the greatest, forget about going for broke and setting your course record. I suggest walking for a set time rather than a specific distance. You expend a great deal of extra energy simply trying to keep yourself upright on snow or ice, so you'll tire more quickly and your typical distance may be more than you can handle. Quality work like intervals, speed, and hills are best left for the treadmill or indoor track.

Let someone know where you're going and the approximate amount of time you'll be gone. Stick to familiar territory and, whenever possible, follow a route that has several safe havens like a corner deli, gas station, or friend's house. A course that loops in a circle is often safer than running to a turn-around and then back again. Loops invariably have you heading toward home.

Of course, during a total whiteout or when the mercury dips to impossibly low depths, it's a good idea to concede defeat and stay indoors. What you're willing to tolerate is a strictly personal thing. (I know some people who need a roof over their heads when the thermometer dips below 49. Yet others would sleep outside in negative number temperatures if their spouses would let them.) On extremely cold days, head for the gym and pound the treadmill rather than the pavement or perhaps get in a little cross-training by doing some other type of cardio exercise. Check out the Wind Chill Factor chart later in this chapter for some stay-indoor guidelines.

Singin' — and walkin' — in the rain

Your tolerance to rain is first and foremost a matter of personal preference. I love exercising in the rain, but I have a friend who swears that one tiny droplet of moisture landing on her skin will melt her like the Wicked Witch of the West. Tolerance to rain is also directly proportional to the temperature. A summer shower can be a welcome respite from the heat, whereas a freezing rain in the dead of winter can quickly take all the joy out of your walk.

A waterproof jacket and pants usually suffice as protection from the rain. Notice that I say waterproof, not water-resistant. Trust me when I tell you that there is a big difference between those two terms. The best rain suits allow the moisture from your perspiration to escape without allowing outside moisture to seep in. I am a big fan of Gore-Tex garments for this purpose.

Though rain in and of itself usually isn't dangerous, thunder and lightning are a different story. I strongly caution you against walking during a thunderstorm, especially out on an open road or field where you are essentially a lightning rod. I once ran a race during a thunderstorm, and it was a frightening experience. Even though I was soaked through to the skin, my hair was standing on end, indicating a buildup of electrical charge and imminent danger of a lightning strike nearby. When I think about it now, I feel angry with myself for risking my life for something as unimportant as finishing a race. Fortunately, no one in the small group of walkers and runners who decided to stick it out and brave the weather was hurt.

The best way to deal with lightning is to avoid it in the first place. If you sense that a thunderstorm is coming, get indoors as quickly as possible. Head for shelter and away from open spaces where you are the tallest target for lightning to strike. If you're hiking or trail walking, don't stay on high points such as peaks and ridges. Crouch low, touching the ground with only your feet to minimize the number of contact points along which electricity can travel. If possible, crouch down on an insulating material such as rope or cloth; stay away from anything metallic. Remove any backpack or clothing that is part metal.

Here's some useful information if you're caught out in a storm: Estimate the distance in miles to a thunderstorm by counting the number of seconds between a flash of lightning and a clap of thunder. Divide this by five to get an estimate of how many miles away the storm is. This number also gives you some idea of how much time you have to hightail it to a safe haven.

When rain combines with dirt, you get mud. During rainy seasons, you get lots of mud. I have nothing good to say about mud. It covers your clothing, spoils your walking shoes, and makes you slip and slide around like a novice ice skater. My only advice: Avoid it at all costs.

Walkin' against the wind

Of all the tricks Mother Nature has up her sleeve, I find wind the most annoying. It slows you down, makes you feel sluggish, and causes you to work harder. Even walking into a light wind of 8 to 10 miles per hour can impede your progress.

You can't do much about the wind except enjoy it when it's at your back. You can wear a windbreaker and pump your arms more vigorously, but those suggestions only help you so much. Perhaps the best idea is to accept wind as a factor like snow and dry sand that slows you down no matter how you slice it. I do recommend using sunblock to minimize windburn and wearing sunglasses to protect your eyes from dust and debris kicked up by a strong gust.

When wind blows across your skin, it removes the insulating layers of warm molecules and replaces them with colder ones. All things being equal, the faster the wind, the greater the heat loss, the colder you feel. Higher winds and lower temperature combine to make the temperature feel colder than it actually is. This is known as *the wind chill factor.*

Table 5-2 shows how wind and temperature correspond to the wind chill factor. Find the wind speed across the top of the chart and the temperature down the left side. These factors meet at the corresponding wind chill factor.

Table 5-2	Wind Chill Factor					
Temperature	**Wind in MPH**					
	5	**10**	**15**	**20**	**25**	**30**
40	37	28	23	19	16	13
35	32	22	16	12	8	6
30	27	16	9	4	1	−2
25	22	10	2	−3	−7	−10
20	16	3	−5	−10	−15	−18
15	11	−3	−11	−17	−22	−25
10	6	−9	−18	−24	−29	−33

Temperature	Wind in MPH					
	5	**10**	**15**	**20**	**25**	**30**
5	0	−15	−25	−31	−36	−44
0	−5	−22	−31	−39	−44	−49
−5	−10	−27	−38	−46	−51	−59
−10	−15	−34	−45	−51	−59	−64
−15	−21	−40	−51	−60	−66	−71
−20	−26	−46	−58	−67	−74	−79

The wind chill factor lets you know whether it's safe for outdoor activities:

Wind chill factor of = − 74 or colder: Extreme danger. Outdoor conditions are dangerous, even for short period of time.

Wind chill factor of = −25 or colder. Unprotected skin can freeze in 1 minute.

Wind chill factor of = −24 or warmer. If you're properly clothed, this shouldn't be a problem.

Part II
Basic Training

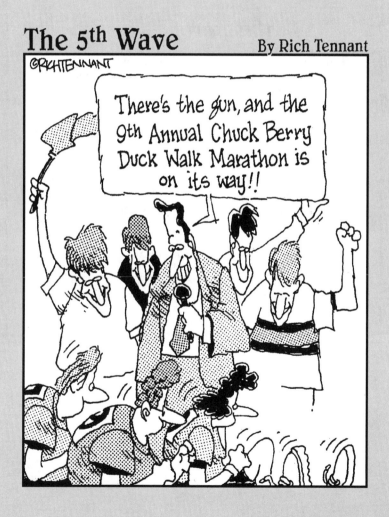

The 5th Wave — By Rich Tennant

There's the gun, and the 9th Annual Chuck Berry Duck Walk Marathon is on its way!!

In this part . . .

This part contains information on the different levels of walking, including some sample routines and workouts for each level. To start this section off, I explain the importance of warming up and cooling down. Then, in the chapters that follow, I explain the different levels of walking. Chapter 7 describes everything you need to know about lifestyle walking, the easiest and lowest-intensity type of walking and the perfect walking technique for beginners. Fitness walking, which I describe in Chapter 8, is the type of walking most walkers do to get in shape. It's a terrific walking technique for burning calories and toning muscles — yet it's easy to do. High-energy walking, an intense style of walking that annihilates calories and works nearly every muscle in your body, is explained in Chapter 9. Chapter 10 covers walk-run and tells you why this is a good way to train if you're interested in combining these two activities for maximum fitness but with minimum risk of injury.

Chapter 6

Warming Up and Cooling Down

● ●

In This Chapter

▶ Understanding the need to warm up before walking

▶ Anatomy of the perfect warm-up

▶ Cooling down for injury prevention

▶ Knowing when to stretch

● ●

*L*ike most people, you probably have a busy life. Though your walking routine is something you enjoy, it requires some dedication and commitment to make the time to get it done. Perhaps that's why you're so tempted to skip the warm-up at the beginning of each walk and the cool-down at the end. You have things to do, so bypassing your warm-up and cool-down can shave valuable minutes off your workout and it won't make a difference. Right? Wrong!

In this chapter, I explain why it's important to make time to ease in and out of your walking workout. I also tell you what constitutes a proper warm-up and cool-down.

The Wisdom of Warming Up

If you've ever tried to start your car on a cold winter's day, you may quickly understand the need for letting your body's engine warm up for a while before you begin your walk. Just as a car feels a little sluggish before its motor has had a chance to idle for a few moments, your body feels a little sluggish when you move from full stop to all-out go without any transition.

The purpose of a warm-up is literally to warm your body up. Raising your body temperature gradually increases the blood flow into your working muscles. It loosens up your muscles, joints, tendons, and ligaments so that you can walk more freely and easily. Warming up makes you less likely to injure yourself because of lack of mobility and flexibility. It also fine-tunes you mentally so that your brain and body are in synch by the time you begin working at a higher level.

The American College of Sports Medicine considers warming up an essential part of any type of workout, even an activity as basic as walking. As a way to transition between rest and exercise, the ACSM — and most walking experts — recommend doing 5-to-10 minutes of some type of slow, repetitive movement that uses the larger muscles of your buttocks, legs, and middle body.

The Perfect Warm-Up

Although a warm-up is crucial, it's not complicated. It can be as simple as walking at a slower-than-workout pace for 5 to 10 minutes before you speed up. I always tell my clients that a warm-up should be done at a trip-over-your-feet-slow pace.

However, some people feel more comfortable doing some other type of activity, like easy cycling or marching in place, as a warm-up. Doing another activity is perfectly acceptable so long as it is slow, easy, and rhythmic and it involves the buttocks, hips, and thigh muscles, the major muscles you use in walking.

I like to use my warm-up as a time for mental prep, too. I try to forget about the thousands of things I need to do that day and focus on the task at hand. What do I want to accomplish during my workout? How does my body feel? Am I up for the full workout I have planned or do I need to make adjustments?

If you're in the first few weeks of your walking program, take the full 10 minutes to warm up. It allows time for your heart, lungs, muscles, and blood vessels to get their juices flowing. My novice walking clients always tell me they feel better, can walk farther and faster, and feel less sore after their workouts when they do a thorough warm-up.

As you get in better shape, you can decrease your warm-up so that it only takes about 5 minutes. But don't ever abandon your warm-up altogether. If you do, you'll miss a valuable opportunity to decrease your risk of injury, ease your muscles into walking, and focus your mind on your workout.

No Time for a Stretch

For some reason, many people think that stretching is an acceptable warm-up activity. This is one of the most prevalent exercise myths I encounter. I can't understand why people aren't getting the message that they should stretch after—rather than before—their workouts.

Stretching before your workout is not a wise idea. In fact, you are more likely to injure yourself by stretching before you warm up because that is when your muscles are the tightest and coldest. Stretching before your muscles are warm and pliable can lead to strains, pulls, and tears.

If you absolutely *must* stretch before you workout, warm up first, stretch for a few moments, and then continue on with the rest of your workout. Or switch to Active Isolated stretching, a technique that combines movement with stretching to raise your body temperature and get your blood flowing and loosen up your muscles. I describe this technique fully in Chapter 12.

Ease On Down the Road

Just as you need to transition into your workout, you need to transition out of it as well. A cool-down has the opposite yet equally essential purpose of your warm-up: It allows time for your body temperature to decrease and allows blood flow to reroute itself from the working muscles back to the rest of your body. You also need that cool-down time to mentally review your workout, set some goals for the workout to follow, and ease out of workout mode.

Once again, the experts at the ACSM have an opinion here. They recommend finishing each workout with a 5-to-10 minute cool-down. I think this is good advice.

Here's a good rule to follow: The more of a novice you are, the longer your cool-down should be. As you get in better shape, you may find that 5 minutes or so is all the cool-down you need.

The Perfect Cool-Down

Your cool-down should be the mirror image of your warm-up. You can walk for 5 to 10 minutes or do another activity at a trip-over-your-feet-slow pace. Include some stretching exercises during this time. Immediately following your slow, easy cool-down, your muscles are warm and very receptive to stretching. As a result, you're less likely to over-stretch or pull a muscle during the cool-down. If you are especially tight, you may appreciate moving your stretch from the beginning to the end of your workout because it may be more comfortable.

An Important Word About Stretching

Ironically, just as people make the mistake of doing their stretching before a workout, many people also make the mistake of heading for the showers after a workout without taking the time to do that all important post-workout stretching. When I said don't stretch at the beginning of your workout, I didn't say forget about it altogether.

Stretching helps maintain flexibility — how far and how comfortably you can move your joints. This is something I discuss in detail in Chapter 12. If you neglect your flexibility, your tendons (the tissues that connect muscle to bone) begin to shorten and tighten. Your movement can become slower and less fluid. You won't be able to stand up as straight, and you may walk more stiffly and with a shorter stride. Doing a full body stretch after each workout can make a big difference in your flexibility.

Flexibility is one of the keys to good walking posture. If your neck muscles are short and tight, your head juts forward. If your shoulders and chest are tight, your shoulders round inward and make it more difficult for you to breathe deeply or use a good strong arm pump. If your lower back, rear thigh, and hip muscles are tight, the curve of your back may become exaggerated, and you may experience back pain, especially as you walk faster. Good flexibility makes your movement more graceful, free, and fluid. It helps eliminate a lot of those aches and pains.

What's more, flexibility exercises can correct muscle imbalances. For instance, suppose that your front thigh muscles are strong, but your rear thighs are tight and weak. (This is a common scenario.) As a result, you end up relying on your front thighs more than you should. Chances are, you won't even notice this, but this imbalance throws off your movement in subtle ways — you may have a short walking stride or bounce too high off the ground. Muscle imbalances can eventually lead to injuries like pulled muscles. They also contribute to clumsiness, which can also lead to injury.

I recommend learning and doing the entire stretching routine that I detail in Chapter 12. It is specially designed for walkers. After completing the stretching routine a couple of times, you may remember how to do the exercises and it should only take you about 5 minutes to complete. Those 5 minutes can go a long way toward helping you walk better, faster, and more comfortably.

Chapter 7

Lifestyle Walking

· ·

· ·

*I*f you can put one foot in front of the other, you're ready to join the ranks of lifestyle walkers. Lifestyle walking doesn't get very complicated, so all you need to do is make just a few tweaks to your basic walking form and posture.

I like to call this beginning level of walking lifestyle walking because it's one of the few forms of exercise that you slip seamlessly into your everyday life without having to make special arrangements. You do this type of walking when you walk around the mall, to the train station, and through the super-market aisles. In other words, it's the type of walking you do to get around in your everyday life. Lifestyle walking requires no special skills or extensive training. You can do it and do it well because you've been doing it all your life. It really is as simple as putting one foot in front of the other.

In fact, lifestyle walking is such a simple activity that you may think it's not worth doing. After all, how much benefit can you get from what is essentially a glorified stroll? As it turns out, a lot.

In recent years, major research studies have found a direct correlation between regular physical activity and improved health. Walking as little as a mile a day at a comfortable pace has been shown to reduce the risk of heart disease, increase stamina, and improve overall health. It has also been shown to reduce stress and fatigue as well as improve self-esteem and mood.

For all these reasons, lifestyle walking is the perfect entry-level exercise activity. In this chapter, I tell you everything you need to know about becoming a lifestyle walker.

Who Is a Lifestyle Walker?

Start your walking program out as a lifestyle walker if most of the following statements apply to you:

- ✔ You have exercised very little, or not at all, in the past 3 months or longer.

- ✔ You answered yes to two or more questions in the section dealing with your risk for heart disease in Chapter 1. If this is the case, check in with your physician before beginning your walking program.

- ✔ You have a body mass index (BMI) of 25 or greater and/or your waist-to-hip ratio is greater than 1 if you are a man or greater than .85 if you are a woman. You can find information on how to determine these measurements in Chapter 1.

- ✔ Your body fat is greater than 20 percent if you're a man or 26 percent if you're a woman. Flip to Chapter 1 to find out how to determine a quick estimate of your body fat percentage.

- ✔ You can't walk a mile at all or can't walk a mile faster than 16:40.

- ✔ Your goals are improved overall health, increased stamina and energy, and modest weight loss.

The Lowdown on Lifestyle Walking

Lifestyle walking is the most casual of walking techniques. It is low to moderate intensity and relatively slow paced. Most lifestyle walkers walk an average of 2.5 to 3.5 miles per hour, which means that they cover 1 mile every 17 to 24 minutes. Your calves, thighs, and hips are the primary muscles used, but you also use your abdominals and lower back to some extent to keep your posture upright. You will feel warm and worked but not sweaty and exhausted when you complete a lifestyle walk.

Because lifestyle walking is the most basic of all walking techniques, beginners can use lifestyle walking to help build stamina and muscular strength. If your goals are weight loss or athletic training, you will probably have to perform more intense exercise than lifestyle walking at some point and work a bit harder at least a few days a week. But if your goals are long-term health and increased stamina to get through your everyday activities, lifestyle walking can remain the foundation of your fitness and exercise program for years to come.

Even if you decide to move beyond lifestyle walking as your primary means of exercise, be sure to review the lifestyle walking techniques and parameters contained in this chapter. You will probably always do some form of lifestyle walking whether you consider it exercise or not. The more activity you do each day, the better. You can also use lifestyle walking to warm up before a more challenging workout and to cool down afterwards.

How much is enough?

The key to successful lifestyle walking is consistency rather than intensity. Although it may seem counterintuitive, lifestyle walkers must walk more frequently than other types of walkers to achieve maximum results. If the bulk of your exercise routine consists of lifestyle walking, I recommend that you walk 30 to 60 minutes most days of the week.

According to recent research, you should aim to burn at least 500 calories through walking each week to improve your health and make noticeable improvements in stamina. You'll see even better gains if you lifestyle walk enough to burn 1,500 calories a week; for most of us, that's an accumulated mileage of about 10 to 20 miles a week. When you walk more than that amount, your health improvement gains are only marginally better.

Contrary to popular belief, you don't have to do all your walking in one shot. You can "collect" walks throughout the day and add them all up. Most experts, including the American College of Sports Medicine, think that several mini-walks are just as beneficial as one long walk. Here are several ways you can achieve your walking goals:

- ✔ Walk once in the morning, once at lunch time, and once after dinner, for a total of three 10- to 20-minute walks.

- ✔ Walk 18 holes around the golf course. For extra calorie burn and exercise, pull your manual golf cart. You'll walk an average of 2 accumulated hours during a round of golf.

- ✔ Walk to the corner store or a friend's house and back for a total of two 20- to 30-minute walks.

- ✔ Window-shop at the mall or your neighborhood shopping district or do your errands on foot to accumulate an hour or more of walking time.

✔ Walk to work, to the train, or to the bus stop. If necessary, get off the train or bus a stop or two early so that you can accumulate two to four 10- to 15-minute walks daily.

✔ Schedule an appointment in your daily planner for a 30- to 60-minute walk on the treadmill or outdoors.

I recommend that you take a twofold strategy to lifestyle walks: Go for a formal lifestyle walk 3 to 6 days a week and squeeze as much "informal" lifestyle walking into your everyday life as you can. Feel free to hit your totals any way you can. Just make sure that your activity level adds up to 30 to 60 minutes of walking most days of the week. If you prefer calorie-related goals, aim to burn 500 to 2,000 calories a week. If you like to focus on mileage, aim for 10 to 20 miles a week.

At this level of walking, you can achieve health benefits. However, most people will probably have to do more than this (and combine their efforts with a healthy, lowfat diet) to achieve significant weight-loss goals. Check out the "Calorie Counter" section in this chapter to estimate the number of calories you burn per minute while lifestyle walking.

My mom is a lifestyle walker. A few days a week she goes to her gym and does a timed 2-mile walk on the treadmill. But the rest of the week she focuses on walking as much as she can during her daily routine. One of her favorite things to do is "aerobic food shopping," which involves zooming through the aisles of the supermarket and grabbing bags, boxes, and bottles as she goes. To do this well, you need a detailed shopping list and a good understanding of the store's layout — otherwise, you're just asking to knock over a display of canned peas!

Determining intensity

Total accrual of miles, minutes, and calories is more important than high intensity in lifestyle walking. Even so, it still makes sense to pay attention to how hard you're working so that you don't overdo it.

I recommend recording your overall exercise intensity in your daily workout log for each walk you do. (I include a sample Walker's Log in Chapter 2.) This record gives you a way to measure your progress. You will find over time that what was hard in the beginning becomes easier as you go along. You can gauge intensity in one of three ways: heart rate, rating of perceived exertion, or the talk test. I describe these techniques in detail in Chapter 5, but here is a brief rundown for reference.

Heart rate

How fast your heart beats correlates directly with how hard you're working. Your target heart rate zone is the range of heart rates that your heart should be beating for a given amount of exercise; it relates to your maximum heart rate. When you are lifestyle walking, strive to be at 50 to 60 percent of your maximum heart rate. This is considered the low end of your training range.

To estimate your maximum heart rate zone, first subtract your age from 220. Then multiply this number by .5 and .6 to come up with your lifestyle walking target heart rate range. For example, if you are 35 years old, you subtract 35 from 220 for an estimated maximum heart rate of 185. When you multiply 185 by .5 and .6, you come up with a range of 93 to 110. Therefore, your heart should be beating 93 to 110 beats per minute when you walk.

You can measure your heart rate, or pulse, at your wrist or the side of your neck. You can use any fingers — except your thumb, which has its own pulse — to take your pulse, but the index and middle fingers are the best fingers to use. You simply count the number of beats you feel in 15 seconds and multiply by 4. Many people prefer to wear a heart rate monitor to avoid doing any math and to get a more accurate measure of heart rate.

Take your heart rate after you've been working out for at least 5 minutes. If you are exercising 30 minutes or more, take your heart rate every 15 to 20 minutes or so. You may also find it useful to take your recovery heart rate, which is your heart rate taken for 1 minute after you stop exercising. The faster your heart rate slows down, the better condition you're in.

Rating of perceived exertion

Some enterprising exercise physiologist in the 1960s came up with a way to quantify how you feel when you're working out. He created a chart called the RPE scale that helps you rate exercise intensity on a scale of 1 to 10. (See the RPE chart in Chapter 5.)

On the RPE scale, 1 represents a level of activity that is really, really easy. You can do it all day without feeling winded. A 1 requires no more effort than sitting in bed, watching TV, and eating popcorn. On the other end of the scale, a 10 represents your maximum level of activity. A 10 feels like you've just run all out for the past hour straight uphill and can't possibly take another step. Obviously, you should strive for a level of activity that falls somewhere in the middle of the scale. For lifestyle walking, an RPE of 4 to 6 is ideal.

The talk test

The talk test is the simplest way to gauge exercise intensity. By talking aloud as you walk, you can tell how hard you're working. If you can sing the latest

Madonna tune at the top of your lungs as you walk along, you aren't working hard enough. If you can't gasp a single syllable, you're working too hard. You should be able to carry on a slightly breathy conversation during a lifestyle walk.

Focus on Form

Just because lifestyle walking can be leisurely and casual doesn't mean form, technique, and posture aren't important. Perfecting posture decreases your chances of injury and soreness. It also lays the groundwork for good posture even when you're not walking.

I like to use a posture checklist as I walk. I start at my head and work my way down, making little corrections along the way. I recommend going through the following checklist once every 10 minutes or so as you walk. You don't want to overthink form, but you do want to reach the point where good posture and walking form are as natural as tying your shoelaces. The woman in Figure 7-1 is demonstrating the proper form for lifestyle walking.

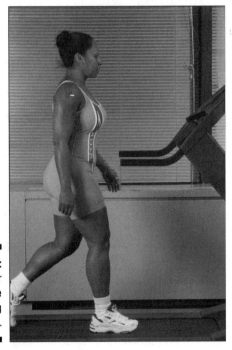

Figure 7-1:
Proper
lifestyle
walking
posture.

Use the following posture-perfect checklist to make sure that your lifestyle walking form is correct:

- ✔ **Head:** Keep your head up and centered between your shoulders. Keep your chin up and focus your eyes straight ahead. Your head and neck should "float" above your shoulders in a relaxed, easy manner.

- ✔ **Shoulders:** Keep them back and down. Don't allow them to round forward or creep up toward your ears.

- ✔ **Chest:** Your chest should be naturally lifted, as if there were a string attached to the center that gently pulls it upwards.

- ✔ **Arms:** Keep your arms low and slightly bent. Swing them easily and naturally.

- ✔ **Hands:** Keep them loosely cupped as if you are holding a butterfly in your hand that you don't want to let escape but you don't want to crush either.

- ✔ **Abdominals:** Pull your belly button gently in toward your spine and tuck your pelvis forward ever so slightly so that you feel tall, stable, and upright. This also protects your lower back.

- ✔ **Hips:** Keep your hips loose and natural. They should move forward and back rather than from side to side.

- ✔ **Thighs:** Your lifestyle walking stride should be natural and unforced, not too long and not too short. Think of your thighs as a link between your hips and your lower legs, assisting both in doing their job.

- ✔ **Feet:** Your heel should strike the ground first, and your toes should gently flex upward. You'll roll heel-arch-ball-toe before completing the step and moving into the next one.

- ✔ **Breathing and heart rate:** Concentrate on keeping your breathing smooth, deep, and regular. If your breathing remains relaxed, your heart will beat rhythmically and steadily.

Lifestyle Walking Routines

Although lifestyle walking can be done anytime, anywhere, having a formal routine to follow helps some walkers. I offer you three different beginner weekly lifestyle walking routines (see Tables 7-1, 7-2, and 7-3) to give you an idea of how easily you can fit lifestyle walking into your day, no matter how busy your schedule is. All three routines get you to the same point: You'll burn the same number of calories, walk the same amount of time, and cover the same miles no matter how you slice it.

To determine how fast you're walking, check out the "Pace finder" sidebar in this chapter.

Table 7-1	Lifestyle Walking Routine 1 — All at Once	
Day 1	Walk 30 to 60 minutes	Intensity: 50 to 60% of max Estimated calorie burn: 120 to 240 Estimated distance: 1.5 to 3.0 miles
Day 2	Walk 30 to 60 minutes	Intensity: 50 to 60% of max Estimated calorie burn: 120 to 240 Estimated distance: 1.5 to 3.0 miles
Day 3	Walk 30 to 60 minutes	Intensity: 50 to 60% of max Estimated calorie burn: 120 to 240 Estimated distance: 1.5 to 3.0 miles
Day 4	REST	
Day 5	Walk 30 to 60 minutes	Intensity: 50 to 60% of max Estimated calorie burn: 120 to 240 Estimated distance: 1.5 to 3.0 miles
Day 6	Walk 30 to 60 minutes	Intensity: 50 to 60% of max Estimated calorie burn: 120 to 240 Estimated distance: 1.5 to 3.0 miles
Day 7	REST	
Weekly Totals	Walking time: 150 to 300 minutes Calories burned: 600 to 1,200 Mileage: 7.5 to 15 miles	

Pace finder

How do you know how fast you're walking? Here's an easy way to figure out your pace. Count the number of steps you take per minute (each time you move your right foot forward).

✔ 60 steps per minute = 2 miles per hour

✔ 90 steps per minute = 3 miles per hour

✔ 100 steps per minute = 3.5 miles per hour

✔ 120 steps per minute = 4 miles per hour

Table 7-2 Lifestyle Walking Routine 2 — Three-Way Split

Day 1	Walk 10 to 20 minutes in the morning. Walk 10 to 20 minutes in the afternoon. Walk 10 to 20 minutes in the evening.	Intensity: 50 to 60% of max Estimated calorie burn: 40 to 80/walk; 120 to 240 daily total Mileage: 0.5 to 1 mile/walk; 1.5 to 3.0 miles daily
Day 2	Walk 10 to 20 minutes in the morning. Walk 10 to 20 minutes in the afternoon. Walk 10 to 20 minutes in the evening.	Intensity: 50 to 60% of max Estimated calorie burn: 40 to 80/walk; 120 to 240 daily total Mileage: 0.5 to 1 mile/walk; 1.5 to 3.0 miles daily
Day 3	Walk 10 to 20 minutes in the morning. Walk 10 to 20 minutes in the afternoon. Walk 10 to 20 minutes in the evening.	Intensity: 50 to 60% of max Estimated calorie burn: 40 to 80/walk; 120 to 240 daily total Mileage: 0.5 to 1 mile/walk; 1.5 to 3.0 miles daily
Day 4	Walk 10 to 20 minutes in the morning. Walk 10 to 20 minutes in the afternoon. Walk 10 to 20 minutes in the evening.	Intensity: 50 to 60% of max Estimated calorie burn: 40 to 80/walk; 120 to 240 daily total Mileage: 0.5 to 1 mile/walk; 1.5 to 3.0 miles daily
Day 5	REST	
Day 6	Walk 10 to 20 minutes in the morning. Walk 10 to 20 minutes in the afternoon. Walk 10 to 20 minutes in the evening.	Intensity: 50 to 60% of max Estimated calorie burn: 40 to 80/walk; 120 to 240 daily total Mileage: 0.5 to 1 mile/walk; 1.5 to 3.0 miles daily
Day 7	REST	
Weekly Totals		Walking time: 150 to 300 minutes Calories burned: 600 to 1,200 weekly Mileage: 7.5 to 15 miles

Table 7-3	Lifestyle Walking Routine 3 — Mix and Match	
Day 1	Walk 30 to 60 minutes.	Intensity: 50 to 60% of max Estimated calorie burn: 120 to 240 Mileage: 1.5 to 3.0 miles
Day 2	Walk 10 to 20 minutes in the morning. Walk 10 to 20 minutes in the afternoon. Walk 10 to20 minutes in the evening.	Intensity: 50 to 60% of max Estimated calorie burn: 40 to 80/walk; 120 to 240 daily total Mileage: .5 to 1 mile/walk; 1.5 to 3.0 miles daily
Day 3	Walk 15 to 30 minutes in the morning. Walk 15 to 30 minutes in the afternoon or evening.	Intensity: 50 to 60% of max Estimated calorie burn: 60 to 120/walk; 120 to 240 daily total Mileage: .75 to 1.5 miles/walk; 1.5 to 3.0 miles daily
Day 4	REST	
Day 5	Walk 30 to 60 minutes.	Intensity: 50 to 60% of max Estimated calorie burn: 120 to 240 Mileage: 1.5 to 3.0 miles
Day 6	Walk 15 to 30 minutes in the morning. Walk 15 to 30 minutes in the afternoon or evening.	Intensity: 50 to 60% of max Estimated calorie burn: 60 to 120/walk; 120 to 240 daily total Mileage: .75 to 1.5 miles/walk; 1.5 to 3.0 miles daily
Day 7	REST	
Weekly Totals	Walking time: 150 to 300 minutes Calories burned: 600 to 1,200 weekly Mileage: 7.5 to 15 miles	

Moving and Improving

Depending on the kind of shape you're in, you may not be able to start out by walking for a full hour, five times a week. In fact, you may not be able to walk for 10 minutes without feeling winded. That's okay. Do what you can: Walk at a pace that's reasonable for you, for the length of time that's comfortable for you, as often as you can.

Your goal should be to work up to doing at least five 30-minute lifestyle walks per week. After you hit this level and can keep up this amount of exercise comfortably for a week or two, gradually increase your time until you can walk a full hour at least 1 or 2 days every week.

If your goal is to simply improve your health, add years to your life, and feel better, then lifestyle walking may be the ultimate walking form for you. In the long run, however, I suspect that most walkers want to move on from doing lifestyle walking as their exclusive form of exercise.

If your aim is to lose weight, build muscle, change the shape of your body, or train for a competition, you will eventually have to move to Level 2 (fitness walking), Level 3 (high-energy walking), or Level 4 (walk-run). But be patient. You can't jump up levels in a matter of days. Typically, if you are starting from scratch, you will spend 4 to 12 weeks building up your fitness base and level of conditioning with lifestyle walking before moving to the next level. When you think that you're ready, redo the evaluations outlined in Chapter 1 and check your score results. Compare them with the information in Chapter 8 to help determine whether you're ready to move on to fitness walking.

Calorie Counter

Use Table 7-4 to determine how many calories you burn during each lifestyle walking workout. Simply look up how many calories you burn per minute based upon your body weight and multiply it by the number of minutes you walk.

Table 7-4	Calories Burned during Lifestyle Walking	
Body Weight (In Pounds)	*Estimated Calorie Burn (Average Speed 3.0 Miles per Hour)*	*Estimated Calorie Burn (Average Speed 3.0 Miles per Hour with Some Modest Hills)*
115 to 125	3 calories/minute	4.5 calories/minute
130 to 140	3.5 calories/minute	5.0 calories/minute
145 to 155	4.0 calories/minute	5.5 calories/minute
160 to 170	4.5 calories/minute	6.0 calories/minute
175 to 185	5.0 calories/minute	6.5 calories/minute
190 to 200	5.5 calories/minute	7.0 calories/minute
205 to 215	6.0 calories/minute	8.0 calories/minute
220 to 230	6.5 calories/minute	8.5 calories/minute
235 to 245	7.0 calories/minute	9.0 calories/minute

Chapter 8

Fitness Walking

• •

In This Chapter

▶ Figuring out whether you're a fitness walker

▶ Defining fitness walking

▶ Concentrating on form and posture

▶ Outlining your fitness walking routines

▶ Intensifying your walking workout

▶ Counting your calories

• •

*M*ost of the people you see walking on a treadmill, a track, or a local jogging path are probably engaging in fitness walking. Fitness walking is the most popular form of walking because, although it's a cinch to do, it's still an effective way to get in serious shape and lose weight. Perhaps that's why more than 70 million people in the U.S. claim to participate in fitness walking on a regular basis.

By picking up the pace, you strengthen your heart and improve aerobic endurance. You strengthen your bones and muscles. You work off stress and improve your moods. You burn lots of calories. And you can accomplish all this with little risk of injury.

Yup. Fitness walking is just about the perfect exercise activity. And in this chapter I give you the info you need to do it.

Who Is a Fitness Walker?

You are ready to try fitness walking if most of the following statements apply to you:

✔ You have been exercising regularly, preferably by lifestyle walking, for the past 6 weeks or more.

✔ You answered yes to one or none of the questions in the section about your risk of heart disease in Chapter 1. If you answered yes to more than one question, first check with your doctor to get the green light to do this moderately strenuous form of exercise.

✔ You have a BMI (body mass index) that is below 25 and/or a waist-to-hip ratio that's less than 1 if you are a man or less than .85 if you are a woman. You can find information on how to determine these measurements in Chapter 1.

✔ Your body fat is between 12 and 20 percent if you're a man or between 16 and 26 percent if you're a woman. Flip to Chapter 1 to find out how to determine a quick estimate of your body fat percentage.

✔ You can walk a mile in less than 15:37 if you're a man or 16:39 if you're a woman.

✔ Your goals are improved overall health, improved muscle tone, and significant weight loss.

Your answers to the above statements should serve as a general guideline — not as hard-and-fast gospel. For instance, even if your BMI is higher than 25 or you can't quite walk a mile as quickly as you should, you may be able to tolerate short periods of fitness walking. And adding some fitness walking to your repertoire will help you get into shape and lose weight faster.

Fitness Walking Defined

Fitness walking is a good way to get in top-notch cardiovascular condition and lose weight. When you fitness walk, you generally move along at a brisk pace of 3.5 to 4.3 miles an hour, covering a mile in a respectable 14 to 17 minutes. Because fitness walking is faster and more intense than lifestyle walking, you work up a sweat and burn significantly more calories.

The extra effort and calorie burn are partly the result of the faster pace. Because you walk faster, you cover more distance in less time. The farther and faster you go, the more calories you burn. Simple as that. But fitness walking is an effective exercise for another reason, too: You use more muscles. Your hips and buttocks get more into the act. And, as a result of your powerful arm swing, so does your upper body. You should see increased overall body tone within 6 to 8 weeks of beginning your fitness walking program.

Most walkers use fitness walking as their main aerobic activity, and indeed, this is a safe and effective workout for a lifetime. Fitness walking is an ideal activity if your goals are longevity, improved health, some improvement in muscle strength and tone, and gradual, moderate weight loss. If you're looking to burn calories at a rate equal to or greater than running, you may want to sprinkle some high-energy walking or walk-run workouts into your routine. Working in some high-energy walking or walk-run workouts is also a good idea if you plan to increase your speed or walk competitively. (Turn to Chapters 9 and 10, respectively, for more about these forms of walking.)

How much is enough?

To strengthen your heart, significantly increase your stamina, and burn a good deal of calories, you must focus on intensity as well as duration in your fitness walking routine. The key is to work your heart and lungs hard enough so that they receive a significant training effect. I discuss how hard is hard enough in the "Determining intensity" section of this chapter.

Strive to fitness walk three to five times a week for 20 to 60 minutes per session. Just as with lifestyle walking (see Chapter 7), you don't have to do your entire walk in one shot. It's okay to split it up into two or three mini-workouts daily.

Ease into a full-fledged fitness walking routine. Don't try to jump in and do 5 full hours a week right off the bat. If you have been building your fitness level with lifestyle walking, start by adding in one or two fitness walking workouts a week. When you can do this easily and without feeling sore or overworked, you can gradually increase your fitness walk frequency to 3 to 5 days a week if you want to.

Just because you begin a fitness walking program doesn't mean that you should abandon lifestyle walking entirely. Even if you don't use lifestyle walking as a formal part of your exercise routine, you should lifestyle walk whenever the opportunity arises, especially if your goal is weight loss. The more you move, the more calories you burn.

Determining intensity

Intensity is a key factor for fitness walking. You are trying to raise your intensity level so that you work up a sweat, give your heart and lungs a good workout, and burn some calories. Track and monitor your walking intensity by taking your heart rate, rating your perceived exertion, or taking the talk test. Although I describe these intensity measuring techniques in detail in Chapter 5, I discuss them briefly here and relate them specifically to fitness walking. Be sure to include a few notes about overall exercise intensity in your workout log so that you can gauge your progress.

Heart rate

How fast your heart beats correlates directly with how hard you're working. When you're fitness walking, you want your target heart rate — the rate at which your heart is beating per minute — to be at 60 to 75 percent of your maximum heart rate, the fastest that your heart is capable of beating.

To estimate your maximum heart rate, subtract your age from 220. Then, multiply this number by .6 and .75 to come up with your fitness walking target heart rate range. For example, if you are 35 years old, subtract 35 from 220 for an estimated maximum heart rate of 185. When you multiply 185 by .6 and .75, you come up with a range of 110 to 140. Therefore, your heart should be beating between 110 and 140 beats per minute when you walk.

You can measure your heart rate, or pulse, at your wrist or the side of your neck. You can use any fingers — except your thumb, which has its own pulse — to take your pulse, but the index and middle fingers are the best fingers to use. You simply count the number of beats you feel in 15 seconds and multiply by 4. You can also strap a heart rate monitor to your chest to get instant and accurate feedback about how quickly your heart is beating at any point during your workout.

Take your heart rate at your peak exercise intensity, meaning at the highest point of your workout. This rate generally occurs in the middle of your workout, when you are walking at the fastest speed of the workout. I also recommend taking your heart rate for 1 minute at the start of your cool-down so that you can gauge how quickly your heart rate recovers. As a general rule, the faster your heart slows down, the better shape you are in.

One of my clients was walking between 3.5 and 4.3 miles an hour with zero percent grade on the treadmill. When we first began tracking his recovery heart rates at the end of his workout, his heart decelerated about 20 beats during the first minute of his cool-down. About 6 weeks after he started his regular fitness walking routine, his heart rate slowed about 40 beats during that first minute of cool-down. In general, the faster your heart rate returns to normal after a workout, the better shape you are in.

Rating of perceived exertion

I give you a detailed description of the rating of perceived exertion (RPE) scale in Chapter 5, but in a nutshell, it is just a quick, easy way to quantify how hard you think you're working out.

The RPE is a scale of 1 to 10, with 1 indicating very easy exercise and 10 indicating very difficult exercise. While you are exercising, think about how your muscles feel, how difficult it is to breath, how much you are sweating, and anything else that contributes to the overall sense of effort. Then assign this effort a number from 1 to 10. Aim for an RPE of between 6 and 8 during your fitness walks.

The talk test

By speaking aloud — even if you don't have anyone to talk to — you can tell how hard you're working. You should be able to offer snatches of breathless conversation during a fitness walk. If you can chatter on about the latest office gossip without stopping for a breath, you need to kick it up a notch. If you can't utter a sound other than gasping for air, you need to slow down.

Focus on Form

If you have been lifestyle walking for the past 6 weeks or more and have really been paying attention to your form, you should have no problem learning the proper fitness walking technique. Your head, shoulder, chest, and abdominal posture remain essentially the same, but you make significant changes to your arm swing and stride to accommodate the faster pace. Essentially, fitness walking is an exaggerated and accelerated form of lifestyle walking.

Thinking through the following head-to-toe checklist becomes even more important when you are fitness walking. Maintaining good form is a bit harder when you're working harder. Many of my clients tell me that their first instinct is to "fall apart" when they begin walking faster because they feel they have to power through any way possible. But good form is more important than moving faster. And if you take the time to perfect your form, you will ultimately walk farther, move faster with greater ease, and reduce your chance of injury. The woman in Figure 8-1 is demonstrating the proper form for fitness walking.

Use the following posture-perfect checklist to make sure that your fitness walking form is correct:

- **Head:** Keep your head up and centered between your shoulders. Keep your chin up and focus your eyes straight ahead. Your head and neck should "float" above your shoulders in a relaxed, easy manner.

- **Shoulders:** Keep them back and down. Don't allow them to round forward or creep up toward your ears.

- **Chest:** Your chest should be naturally lifted, as if a string were attached to the center that gently pulls it upward.

- **Arms:** Your arms should be bent at 90 degrees. Swing them back and forth — not side to side — and keep them close to your body. At the top of your arm swing, your elbow will be level with your breastbone; at the bottom of your swing, your hand will brush your hip.

- **Hands:** Keep them loosely cupped as if you are holding a butterfly in your hand that you don't want to let escape but that you don't want to crush either.

✔ **Abdominals:** Pull your belly button gently in toward your spine and tuck your pelvis forward ever so slightly so that you feel tall, stable, and upright. This also protects your lower back.

✔ **Hips:** Power your movements from your hips rather than your thighs, but keep your hips loose and natural. They should move forward and back rather than from side to side.

✔ **Thighs:** Take short, fast strides that still feel natural rather than awkward.

✔ **Feet:** Land firmly on your heel and roll smoothly to push off with the toes. Think of planting your heel and then "pushing the ground away from you" as you roll through your foot.

✔ **Breathing and heart rate:** Your breathing will be loud, but concentrate on keeping it even and steady. Your heart will be thumping, but focus on keeping the beats steady and regular.

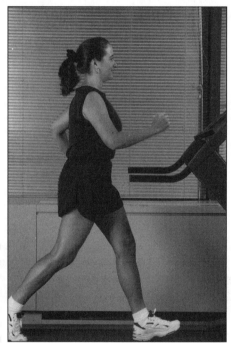

Figure 8-1:
Proper
fitness
walking
form.

As you move through the posture checklist, keep in mind these common form mistakes. Many of the following bad habits may have been ingrained in you since childhood, so it may take some effort and deep thinking on your part to correct them. But the results will be worth it. You'll look better, get fewer aches and pains, and burn more calories because you'll be able to go farther, faster.

✔ **Rocking the baby:** Holding your arms up too high and swinging them from side to side, as shown in Figure 8-2, is known as "rocking the baby" because it looks like you're rocking a baby to sleep. Concentrate on relaxing your shoulders and lowering your arms. Make sure that you have no more than a 90-degree bend at the elbows.

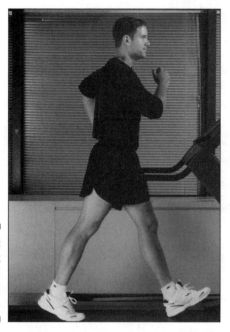

Figure 8-2: Don't "rock the baby" when you walk.

✔ **Bubble butt:** You make your butt appear bigger when you overarch your lower back and stick your buttocks out. This form can cause strain to your lower back and even your knees because it tends to make you lock your knees as you walk. To counteract bubble butt syndrome, demonstrated in Figure 8-3, make sure that your abs are pulled in tight and that you tuck your pelvis under ever so slightly.

✔ **Pounder feet:** If your foot makes a loud slap when it strikes the ground, you aren't rolling through your entire foot. In this case, concentrate on lifting your toe as you step out, striking heel first as your foot makes contact with the ground, and then rolling through the entire length of the foot before moving into the next stride.

✔ **Shuffle feet:** If you tend to trip over your feet a lot, you aren't picking them up high enough, and you are spending too much time on the balls of your feet and toes. The correction is the same as for pounder feet.

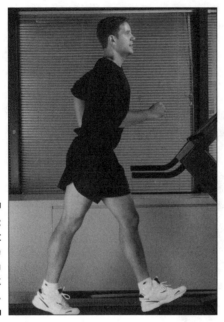

Figure 8-3:
Bubble butt
syndrome
can strain
your back
and knees.

✔ **Turkey strut:** When you allow your head to fall forward and your chin to jut out, it gives you the look of a turkey (see Figure 8-4). Concentrate on keeping your head between your shoulders, your chest lifted, and your shoulders square and relaxed.

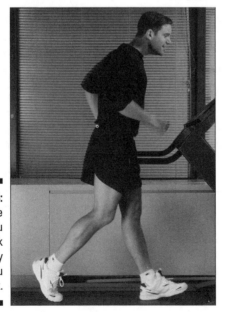

Figure 8-4:
Make sure
that you
don't look
like a turkey
when you
walk.

Fitness Walking Routines

The fitness walking routines in Tables 8-1, 8-2, and 8-3 take a 9-week ramped approach to your workouts. The first routine adds a few fitness walks into your workouts; it's ideal for those just working into higher level exercise. The second routine adds 1 additional fitness walking day per week, and the third routine has you fitness walking 5 days a week. Do the first routine for a week or two and then, if you feel comfortable, ramp up to the second routine and then the third.

This gradual approach helps you increase your fitness routine without inviting injury. I know that being patient when exercising and burning calories is hard, but try to take a long-range view of the shape-up process: You can use this routine for the rest of your life. You can view this increase in terms of the number of calories you burn, the amount of mileage you cover, or the amount of time you spend walking.

Note that as you add in fitness walk workouts, you actually spend less time exercising but burn more calories. Pretty good deal, huh?

Table 8-1	Fitness Walking Routine 1 — Weeks 1–3	
Day 1	Lifestyle walk 30 to 60 minutes	Intensity: 50 to 60% of max Estimated calorie burn: 120 to 240 Estimated distance: 1.5 to 3.0 miles
Day 2	Fitness walk 30-45 minutes	Intensity: 60 to 75% of max Estimated calorie burn: 180 to 270 Estimated distance: 1.9 to 3.0 miles
Day 3	Lifestyle walk 30 to 60 minutes	Intensity: 50 to 60% of max Estimated calorie burn: 120 to 240 Estimated distance: 1.5 to 3.0 miles
Day 4	REST	
Day 5	Fitness walk 30 to 45 minutes	Intensity: 60 to 75% of max Estimated calorie burn: 180 to 270 Estimated distance: 1.9 to 3.0 miles
Day 6	Lifestyle walk 30 to 60 minutes	Intensity: 50 to 60% of max Estimated calorie burn: 120 to 240 Estimated distance: 1.5 to 3.0 miles
Day 7	REST	
Weekly Totals	Walking time: 150 to 270 minutes Calories burned: 720 to 1,260 Mileage: 8.3 to 15 miles	

Table 8-2	Fitness Walking Routine 2 — Weeks 4–6	
Day 1	Lifestyle walk 30 to 60 minutes	Intensity: 50 to 60% of max Estimated calorie burn: 120 to 240 Estimated distance: 1.5 to 3.0 miles
Day 2	Fitness walk 30 to 45 minutes	Intensity: 60 to 75% of max Estimated calorie burn: 180 to 270 Estimated distance: 1.9 to 3.0 miles
Day 3	Fitness walk 30 to 45 minutes	Intensity: 60 to 75% of max Estimated calorie burn: 180 to 270 Estimated distance: 1.9 to 3.0 miles
Day 4	Lifestyle walk 30 to 60 minutes	Intensity: 50 to 60% of max Estimated calorie burn: 120 to 240 Estimated distance: 1.5 to 3.0 miles
Day 5	REST	
Day 6	Fitness walk 30 to 45 minutes	Intensity: 60 to 75% of max Estimated calorie burn: 180 to 270 Estimated distance: 1.9 to 3.0 miles
Day 7	REST	
Weekly Totals	Walking time: 150 to 255 minutes Calories burned: 780 to 1,290 weekly Mileage: 8.7 to 15 miles	

Table 8-3	Fitness Walking Routine 3 — Weeks 7–9	
Day 1	Fitness walk 30 to 45 minutes	Intensity: 60 to 75% of max Estimated calorie burn: 180 to 270 Estimated distance: 1.9 to 3.0 miles
Day 2	Fitness walk 30 to 45 minutes	Intensity: 60 to 75% of max Estimated calorie burn: 180 to 270 Estimated distance: 1.9 to 3.0 miles
Day 3	Fitness walk 30 to 45 minutes	Intensity: 60 to 75% of max Estimated calorie burn: 180 to 270 Estimated distance: 1.9 to 3.0 miles
Day 4	REST	
Day 5	Fitness walk 30 to 45 minutes	Intensity: 60 to 75% of max Estimated calorie burn: 180 to 270 Estimated distance: 1.9 to 3.0 miles

Day 6	Fitness walk 30 to 45 minutes	Intensity: 60 to 75% of max Estimated calorie burn: 180 to 270 Estimated distance: 1.9 to 3.0 miles
Day 7	REST	
Weekly Totals	Walking time: 150 to 225 minutes Calories burned: 900 to 1,350 weekly Mileage: 9.5 to 15 miles	

Moving and Improving

Fitness walking will probably form the basis of a walking exercise program for most people, but lifestyle walking can still play an important part in your health efforts. Remember, the more you move, the more you lose! If a combination of fitness and lifestyle walking meets your goals and you feel good doing them, you don't need to push yourself harder. However, you may want to walk at a higher intensity for a variety of reasons.

Higher intensity walking can help you accelerate weight loss, increase muscle mass, or prepare for competitive walks. You may just like the feel of the wind whipping through your hair. If so, you can integrate other types of walking or cross-training activities into your cardiovascular repertoire. Here are some ways to boost your walking workouts:

✔ Do 1 to 2 days a week of high-energy walking (Chapter 9).

✔ Do 1 to 2 days a week of walk-run (Chapter 10).

✔ Do 1 to 2 days a week of interval training (Chapter 13).

✔ Do 1 to 2 days a week of fitness walking up and down hills (Chapter 17).

Remember not to overdo high-intensity training, especially if you're new to the speed game. Doing too much too soon leaves you sore and sets you up for injuries. Spend at least 9 weeks doing the fitness walking routine outlined in the tables earlier in this chapter. This routine gives you a firm base of mileage and lung power to work with. When you think you're ready to move onward and upward, redo the evaluations outlined in Chapter 1 and check your score results. Compare your results with the information in Chapter 9 to help you determine whether you're ready to move on to high-energy walking. I also encourage you to explore some of the other advanced walking techniques that I outline throughout this book.

Calorie Counter

Use Table 8-4 to determine how many calories you burn during each workout. Simply look up how many calories you burn per minute based upon your body weight and multiply it by the number of minutes you walk.

Table 8-4	Calories Burned during Fitness Walking	
Body Weight (In Pounds)	**Estimated Calorie Burn (Average Speed 3.75 Miles per Hour)**	**Estimated Calorie Burn (Average Speed 3.75 Miles per Hour with Some Modest Hills)**
115 to 125	4 calories/minute	6 calories/minute
130 to 140	4.5 calories/minute	6.5 calories/minute
145 to 155	5.0 calories/minute	7.0 calories/minute
160 to 170	5.5 calories/minute	8.0 calories/minute
175 to 185	6.0 calories/minute	8.5 calories/minute
190 to 200	7.0 calories/minute	9.0 calories/minute
205 to 215	7.5 calories/minute	9.5 calories/minute
220 to 230	8.0 calories/minute	10.0 calories/minute
235 to 245	8.5 calories/minute	10.5 calories/minute

Chapter 9

High-Energy Walking

. . . .

In This Chapter

▶ Deciding whether you're ready for high-energy walking

▶ Understanding high-energy walking

▶ Working on your walking form

▶ Selecting a high-energy walking routine

▶ Walking off the calories

▶ Entering the "gray zone"

. . . .

My high school track team had one race walker. She was good — good enough to compete at the national level. Even so, the other track athletes used to tease her. In those days, it was bizarre to see someone walking with an exaggerated wiggle of the hips, arms pumping furiously, striding along in an unwavering straight line as if she were balanced on a high wire. Yeah, we made fun of her, but she never got injured — as many of the runners on the team did — and her walking speeds were nearly as fast as many of our teammate's running speeds. It was only years later, when the popularity of race walking and speed walking exploded, that I realized that the girl we used to poke friendly fun at was onto something.

I refer to the version of speed walking in this book as high-energy walking. If you're looking for a fast, furious, fun way to burn more calories and work more muscles than any other style of walking, high-energy walking is made for you. In fact, you'll burn almost as many calories as you do while running — and in some cases more! But because it's still a form of walking, you get high-impact results from a low-impact activity, so your risk of injury is still minimal.

High-energy walking — a version of speed walking — is an excellent activity for anyone who seeks high-level aerobic and total body conditioning. In this chapter, I give you the skinny on high-energy walking, explaining everything from proper technique to injury prevention.

Are You Ready for High-Energy Walking?

You're ready to try high-energy walking if most of the following statements apply to you:

- ✔ You have been exercising regularly and have done at least one fitness walk or walk-run a week for the past 6 weeks or more.

- ✔ You answered yes to one or none of the questions in the section dealing with your risk for heart disease in Chapter 1. If you answered yes to two or more questions, first check with your doctor to get the green light to do this moderate-to-challenging strenuous form of exercise.

- ✔ You have a BMI (body mass index) that is between 18.5 and 25 and/or a waist-to-hip ratio less than 1 if you are a man or less than .85 if you are a woman. You can find information on how to determine these measures in Chapter 1.

- ✔ Your body fat is between 12 and 20 percent if you're a man or between 16 and 26 percent if you're a woman. Flip to Chapter 1 to find out how to determine a quick estimate of your body fat percentage.

- ✔ You can walk a mile in less than 15:37 if you are a man or 16:39 if you are a woman.

- ✔ You have few, if any, chronic joint problems, such as knee, ankle, hip, or lower back discomfort.

- ✔ Your goals are increased speed, optimal endurance, maximum muscle usage, and excellent weight loss results, and/or you are training for a competition.

- ✔ You are a runner who wants to enhance or supplement your running program, and/or you are looking for an activity that offers similar results to running.

Your answers to the above statements should serve as a general guideline. You can try high-energy walking even if you can't walk quite as fast as the paces listed above. In fact, high-energy walking is a way to develop speed and endurance. If you've been thinking about trying out a running program but are concerned about developing or exacerbating joint problems, high-energy walking can be a satisfactory activity, giving even hard-core speed junkies a run for their money.

High-Energy Walking Defined

High-energy walking is a version of race walking. The difference is that you may not walk as fast or wiggle your hips quite as much as a race walker does when you do high-energy walking. It is an unparalleled aerobic conditioning activity, offering similar calorie burns and weight loss potential as a running program, yet it's much easier on the body than running. When you high-energy walk, you generally move along at a lightning-fast pace of 4.4 to 6.0 miles an hour, covering a mile in a blazing time of 10 to 13.6 minutes.

Just one look at high-energy walkers, with their wiggling hips and quick linear stride, confirms that high-energy walking uses more muscles than any other type of walking. The extra effort and calorie burn are partly the result of moving at a faster pace as well. Because you walk faster, you cover more distance in less time. The farther you go, the more calories you burn.

Some scientists speculate that high-energy walking burns 1.5 to 2 times as many calories as other types of walking over the same distance because of the extra muscle involvement and effort expended. That's a calorie burn similar to running for the same amount of time. You also tone your muscles for a sleeker body shape — high-energy walking exercises the buttocks, thighs, hips, shoulders, upper back, and abs. You probably will see a marked increase in tone and a decrease in body fat within 6 to 8 weeks of adding one to three high-energy walks a week into your overall walking program.

Most walkers use high-energy walking as a "hard day" aerobic activity, not their everyday workout. High-energy walking a few times a week is a great way to kick your fitness level up a notch. Some walkers get addicted to the speed of high-energy walking and eventually use it as their primary cardio workout. That's okay, provided that you use good form and don't experience burnout or injury as a result.

Some extremely ambitious high-energy walkers advance to the next level by entering road races in the race walking division. This is a small but growing sport. And I have long since learned not to underestimate race walkers. I remember running a 10K race once and having a race walker blow right past me. Being outrun by a walker was a humbling experience.

If you are interested in competitive race walking, I recommend checking with your local running or walking club to see whether it has a race walking division or offers any race walking instruction. Because race walking is a very precise activity, some initial coaching to understand the basics can be extremely helpful. You can visit www.racewalk.com to find a list of race walking clubs and references in your area.

How much is enough?

The key to high-energy walking is form and speed. The better your form, the faster you'll be able to move. The faster you move, the more benefits you'll derive from your high-energy walking workouts.

Add one to three high-energy walks a week into your routine if you are looking to build speed or burn a lot of calories. Each high-energy workout should last from 20 to 60 minutes, including your warm-up and cool-down at an easier pace. Competitive walkers may want to do four to five high-energy workouts a week.

Mastering high-energy walking takes time, so be sure to review the "Focus on Form" section and the posture checklist later in this chapter before you jump into a full-fledged high-energy walking program. Slower is better in the beginning because you have an easier time correcting your form when you're not trying to zip along at the speed of light. If you have been building your fitness level with lifestyle and fitness walking, start by adding in one high-energy walking workout a week. After you can do this easily and without feeling sore or overworked, you can gradually increase your high-energy walking frequency to 3 to 5 days a week if you want to.

Determining intensity

High-energy walking is the most challenging type of walking I discuss in this book. Carefully monitor your intensity level to make sure that you get into the proper training range and don't go overboard. Track and monitor your walking intensity by taking your heart rate, determining your rating of perceived exertion, or taking the talk test. Although I describe these ways of measuring your intensity in detail in Chapter 5, I discuss them briefly in this section and relate them specifically to high-energy walking. Include a few notes about overall exercise intensity in your workout log so that you can gauge your progress.

Heart rate

How fast your heart beats correlates directly with how hard you're working. During high-energy walking, you want your target heart rate — the rate at which your heart is beating per minute — to be at 75 to 95 percent of your *maximum heart rate,* the fastest that your heart is capable of beating.

High-energy walking is done at an extremely high intensity, so be sure that you put in your training time before you attempt to do this on a regular basis. Otherwise, you're asking for a blowout injury or extreme muscle soreness for days after such a high-intensity workout.

To estimate your maximum heart rate zone, subtract your age from 220. Then multiply this number by .75 and .95 to come up with your high-energy walking target heart rate range. For example, if you are 35 years old, subtract 35 from 220 for an estimated maximum heart rate of 185. When you multiply 185 by .75 and .95, you come up with a range of 140 to 175. Therefore, your heart should be beating 140 to 175 beats per minute when you walk.

You can measure your heart rate, or pulse, at your wrist or the side of your neck. You can use any fingers — except your thumb, which has its own pulse — to take your pulse, but the index and middle fingers are the best fingers to use. You simply count the number of beats you feel in 15 seconds and multiply by 4. You can also strap a heart rate monitor to your chest to get instant and accurate feedback about how quickly your heart is beating at any point during your workout.

Take your heart rate at your peak exercise intensity, which gives you the highest rate of your workout. You generally reach this peak rate in the middle of your workout, when you are walking at the fastest speed of the workout. I also recommend taking your heart rate for 1 minute shortly after you begin your cool-down so that you can gauge how quickly your heart rate recovers. As a general rule, the faster your heart slows down, the better shape you are in.

If you are really serious about your high-energy walking workouts, I recommend getting your true maximum heart rate measured by a physician or qualified trainer. The age-predicted method of determining heart rate that I give you throughout this book is really just an estimation of maximum heart rate based on extrapolations of various studies down over the years. This number can be off by as much as 30 beats per minute. This reading doesn't really affect you too much until you strive to stay in the upper regions of your target training range.

Your true maximum heart rate is the fastest your heart is able to beat even if you are given more work. You can find out your true maximum heart rate by taking a sub-maximal stress test, which is usually performed on a stationary bike or treadmill. You ride, walk, or run at an ever-increasing pace until continuing becomes too difficult. During your stress test, your physician or trainer is measuring your heart rate and other physical parameters. Depending on how sophisticated a setup your doctor or trainer has access to, you may be hooked up to a series of electrodes and an oxygen analyzer gas mask.

Rating of perceived exertion

I give you a detailed description of the rating of perceived exertion (RPE) scale in Chapter 5, but essentially, it is just a quick, easy way to quantify how hard you think you're working out. You take into account everything from the way your muscles feel to how hard you're breathing and assign it a number that correlates with the level of difficulty you're working at.

The RPE is a scale of 1 to 10, with 1 indicating very easy exercise and 10 indicating very difficult exercise. You assign your perceived sense of effort a number from 1 to 10. During your high-energy walks, aim for an RPE of between 8 and 10.

The talk test

By speaking aloud — even if you don't have anyone to talk to — you can tell how hard you're working. You should barely be able to speak during the peak of your high-energy walking workouts, but you should be able to throw out a breathless word or two here or there. If you can chatter comfortably, pick up the pace. If you feel like you're gasping for air and you can't sputter a single word because you're working so hard, slow it down a touch.

Focus on Form

Most people think that to walk faster you should lengthen your stride, but that isn't true. The secret to high-energy walking form is taking more steps per minute at your normal or a slightly shorter-than-normal stride. Imagine that you're on a tightrope so that one stride lines up directly in front of the other. Don't swing out to the side like you do in other forms of walking. This technique results in the patented high-energy walking hip wiggle that's similar to a race walker's form.

In high-energy walking, your feet follow your arms. In other words, you use your arms to propel your body forward. If you swing your arms in a straight-forward and confident manner and focus on matching your stride to your arms' movement, you'll walk faster and straighter.

Style is the most important factor when you first start practicing high-energy walking. When you first try it, the hip roll will feel a bit cartoonish, and the stride will feel forced. You may need two to three workouts to feel totally comfortable. Concentrate more on your style than how fast you walk until you are sure that you have perfected your technique. Thinking through your head-to-toe, posture-perfect checklist can help you understand the characteristics of high-energy walking. After you master this walking form, you'll feel like you're skimming along, your feet barely touching the surface of the ground. The man in Figure 9-1 is demonstrating proper high-energy walking form.

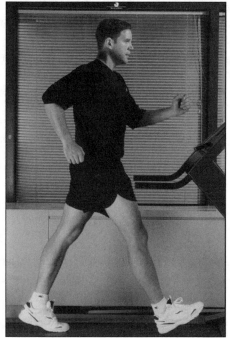

Figure 9-1:
Proper
high-energy
walking
posture.

Use the following posture-perfect checklist to make sure that your high-energy walking form is correct:

✔ **Head:** Keep your head up and centered between your shoulders. Keep your chin up and focus your eyes straight ahead. Your head and neck should "float" above your shoulders in a relaxed, easy manner.

✔ **Shoulders:** Keep them back and down. Don't allow them to round forward or creep up toward your ears.

✔ **Chest:** Your chest should be naturally lifted, as if a string were attached to the center that gently pulls it upward.

✔ **Arms:** Your arms should be bent at slightly less than 90 degrees. Swing them back and forth — not side to side — like a pendulum and keep them close to your body. At the top of the arm swing, your elbow will be level with your breastbone; at the bottom of the arm swing, your hand will brush your hip. Swing your arms briskly and definitely.

✔ **Hands:** Keep them loosely cupped as if you are holding a butterfly in your hand that you don't want to let escape but you don't want to crush either.

✔ **Abdominals:** Lean forward slightly so that you feel as if you are "tumbling with control" as you walk forward. Pull your belly button gently in toward your spine to help protect your lower back.

✔ **Hips:** Because your stride is quick and linear, move your hips in a sort of exaggerated wiggle. Use your hips to propel you forward so that you walk at a fast rate.

✔ **Thighs:** Take more steps per minute at your normal or a slightly shorter-than-normal stride length. Straighten the advancing leg so that your knee is fairly straight from the moment of first contact with the ground until you are just about to swing forward with your other leg.

✔ **Feet:** Imagine that you are walking along a tightrope. Each footfall should land squarely on the imaginary line directly in front of you so that you don't stray from walking in a straight line. Get a good toe lift by using your ankles. Land heel first, roll through the foot, and then push off firmly and vigorously. Your footfall should match the rhythm of your arm swing.

✔ **Breathing and heart rate:** Your breathing will be deep and strong, but try to keep it regular and steady. Your heart will be pounding, but focus on staying relaxed.

High-energy walking requires practice to get the technique down right. Here are some exercises you can do to help you get the feel of certain aspects of high-energy form.

✔ **Forward lean:** Walk at a slow pace for a few minutes, first exaggerating your forward lean and then exaggerating your backward lean. Notice how your body feels in each position. Now walk with an ever-so-slight lean forward. You should observe a definite driving sensation as you reach out with your lead leg. Once you feel this sensation, gradually speed up until you can feel it while walking at full high-energy throttle.

✔ **Back and abdomen:** Many people stick their butts out when they high-energy walk, a posture that can lead to lower back pain. This poor posture is often due to tight lower back muscles and weak abdominal muscles that don't have the ability to sustain proper posture. To counteract weakness, check out Chapter 11 for the partial roll up and opposite extensions exercises. To counteract tightness, check out Chapter 12 for the cat-cow, pretzel, and knee hug stretches.

✔ **Shoulder and arm action:** Try the following mental imagery to help you hold your shoulders and swing your arms correctly. Think of your spine as a stationary pole with your body rotating around it. Because this rod allows only a fixed path, you cannot twist from side to side or swing your arms across your body. Practice correct and incorrect arm movements in front of a mirror so that you can see the difference. If you have access to a treadmill near a mirror, you can do this exercise while actually moving.

✔ **Hip action:** The most common cause of improper hip action is poor flexibility. Do the pretzel and knee hug stretches listed in Chapter 12 to help improve hip flexibility. It helps to imagine two stripes running down the front of your legs. When you are using correct hip action, these stripes will move forward and back in relation to the vertical line of your body rather than from side to side.

- ✔ **Thigh action:** Try to land as close as possible to your other foot to avoid overreaching your stride. Emphasize your toe lift. Warm up thoroughly before moving into a full-blown high-energy walk so that you have the flexibility to move your knees and hips properly.

- ✔ **Foot and ankle action:** Focus on keeping your toes pointed forward without any splay inward or outward. Try walking on your heels with your toes up off the ground for a few minutes. Incorporate this exercise into your pre-walk warm-up. Stretch your calves and shins immediately after each high-energy walk workout. (Turn to Chapter 12 for some stretching exercises.)

High-Energy Walking Routines

In this section I give you three simple high-energy walking workouts to try. They are designed for walkers who want to add one to two high-energy walks a week into their current walking program.

The first program (Table 9-1) is an interval-type training program: It alternates periods of fitness walking with periods of high-energy walking. I recommend that you start with this workout first to give your body a chance to adjust to this very different and strenuous walking style. After a few weeks, try the second full-fledged high-energy routine.

Table 9-1	High-Energy Walking Routine 1	
Interval	*Walking Level*	*Total Time*
Warm-up	Lifestyle walking	5 minutes
1	Fitness walking	3 minutes
2	High-energy walking	2 minutes
3	Fitness walking	3 minutes
4	High-energy walking	2 minutes
5	Fitness walking	3 minutes
6	High-energy walking	2 minutes
7	Fitness walking	2 minutes
8	High-energy walking	3 minutes
9	Fitness walking	2 minutes
Cool-down	Lifestyle walking	5 minutes
Total walking time		32 minutes

The second high-energy walk workout (Table 9-2) is a go-for-broke high-energy walk. You may want to try this on a track or a treadmill at first so that you don't have to worry about surface inconsistencies. You have an easier time keeping track of your pace on a track or treadmill because most tracks measure a quarter of a mile and most treadmills are equipped with a feature that displays the time and distance that you've walked.

Table 9-2	High-Energy Walking Routine 2	
Interval	*Walking Level*	*Total Time*
Warm-up	Lifestyle walking	5 minutes
1	Fitness walking	3 minutes
2	High-energy walking	15 to 44 minutes
3	Fitness walking	3 minutes
Cool-down	Lifestyle walking	5 minutes
Total walking time		31 to 60 minutes

The third high-energy walk workout (Table 9-3) takes a somewhat different approach than most of the workouts in this book. I based it on distance traveled rather than time of intervals. I developed this workout with competitive walkers in mind because many competitive athletes base their goals on distances traveled rather than total exercise time. Once again, I recommend trying this workout on a track or treadmill to more accurately gauge your distances.

Table 9-3	High-Energy Walking Routine 3	
Interval	*Walking Level*	*Total Distance*
Warm-up	Lifestyle walking	0.25 miles
1	Fitness walking	0.25 miles
2	High-energy walking	0.50 miles
3	Fitness walking	0.25 miles
4	High-energy walking	0.50 miles
5	Fitness walking	0.25 miles
6	High-energy walking	1.0 miles
7	Fitness walking	0.25 miles

Interval	Walking Level	Total Distance
8	High-energy walking	0.75 miles
9	Fitness walking	0.25 miles
Cool-down	Lifestyle walking	0.25 miles
Total walking distance		4.50 miles

Calorie Counter

Use Table 9-4 to determine how many calories you burn during each workout. Simply look up how many calories you burn per minute based upon your body weight and multiply it by the number of minutes you walk.

Table 9-4	Calories Burned during High-Energy Walking	
Body Weight (In Pounds)	**Estimated Calorie Burn (Average Speed 4.75 Miles per Hour)**	**Estimated Calorie Burn (Average Speed 4.75 Miles per Hour with a Few Modest Hills)**
115 to 125	7 calories/minute	8 calories/minute
130 to 140	8 calories/minute	9 calories/minute
145 to 155	8.5 calories/minute	10 calories/minute
160 to 170	9.5 calories/minute	11 calories/minute
175 to 185	10 calories/minute	12 calories/minute
190 to 200	11 calories/minute	13 calories/minute
205 to 215	12 calories/minute	14 calories/minute
220 to 230	13 calories/minute	14.5 calories/minute
235 to 245	13.5 calories/minute	15.5 calories/minute

Welcome to the Gray Zone

When you walk at speeds so fast that breaking into a run would be easier, your calorie burn increases exponentially. Scientists refer to this supersonic walking pace as the gray zone. For most people, this gray zone is somewhere between 5.0 and 6.0 miles per hour, depending on your leg length, body mechanics, and fitness level. Studies have shown that holding yourself to a walk rather than running can burn calories equal to fast running — up to 400 calories in 30 minutes for a person weighing approximately 135 pounds.

If you're looking to burn mega-calories, try a 20-minute gray zone walk. Gray zone walking is like a revved-up version of high-energy walking: You take short, quick, decisive strides. But to get into the gray zone, you have to walk so fast that you are holding yourself back from transitioning into a trot. Maintain tall posture, keep your shoulders relaxed, and hold your arms slightly above parallel to the ground as you swing them in opposition to your feet. Don't swing your arms across your body or you won't be able to build enough momentum to move as fast as you need to. Power your leg movements from your hips so that your hips and rear move in a slightly exaggerated wiggle. When you combine gray zone walking with a 5-minute warm-up and a 5-minute cool-down, you burn about 330 calories. (You may burn more or fewer calories depending upon your weight.)

Chapter 10

Walk-Run

● ●

In This Chapter

▶ Determining whether walk-run is for you

▶ Citing the benefits of walk-run

▶ Knowing how hard to go

▶ Perfecting your running form

▶ Picking out a walk-run routine

▶ Working off the calories

▶ Figuring out your pace and speed

● ●

*R*unning has always had an elitist reputation. Many of my new clients tell me that running is the only exercise that ever gets them into shape. When I recommend that my clients start with walking, I often see the skepticism in their eyes. When I tell them that they can stick with walking and gain top-notch fitness without ever running a step, they really think I'm nuts. They just don't believe that walking can get them into shape.

Because some walkers do feel that they want to run at least some of the time, I dedicate this entire chapter to an activity known as walk-run. Walk-run is exactly what it sounds like: a workout in which you alternate walking and running. In fact, walk-run is gaining popularity among exercisers and is becoming a phenomenon in its own right. A few companies, notably Nike and Side1, even make a special shoe designed for those who walk-run.

If you are interested in trying walk-run, this chapter tells you everything you need to know about safely including it in your routine. However, walk-run is an *optional* walking workout. If you never so much as break into a jog, you can still get into great shape by exercising at all other levels of walking and with other types of workouts described throughout this book. However, you may want to try walk-run because it's fun and because it's another way to add variety to your workouts.

Who Should Try Walk-Run?

You're ready to try walk-run if most of the following statements apply to you:

✔ You have been exercising regularly and have done at least one high-energy walk a week for the past 6 weeks or more.

✔ You answered yes to one or none of the questions in the section about your risk for heart disease in Chapter 1. If you answered yes to two or more questions, check with your doctor to get the green light to do this moderate-to-challenging strenuous form of exercise.

✔ You have a BMI (body mass index) between 18.5 and 25 and/or a waist-to-hip ratio less than 1 if you are a man or less than .85 if you are a woman. You can find information on how to determine these measurements in Chapter 1.

✔ Your body fat is between 12 and 20 percent if you're a man or between 16 and 26 percent if you're a woman. Flip to Chapter 1 to find out how to determine a quick estimate of your body fat percentage.

✔ You can walk a mile in less than 15:37 if you're a man or 16:39 if you're a woman.

✔ You have few, if any, chronic joint problems, such as knee, ankle, hip, or lower back discomfort.

✔ Your goals are increased speed, optimal endurance, maximum muscle usage, and excellent weight loss results, and/or you are training for a competition.

✔ Your goal is to begin a running program or use running as a cross-training activity on a regular basis.

Your answers to the above statements are only a general guideline. So even if you can't walk a mile as speedily as the above guidelines recommend, there's no reason why you can't toss a few minutes of light trotting into your program. Use your judgment; only you can determine whether you're ready to add jogging and running intervals into your walking repertoire. You may find that you like the feeling of moving at a different gait once in a while, especially if it doesn't leave you feeling overworked and you're not prone to injury. (For more information about running, check out *Running For Dummies,* by Florence "Flo-Jo" Griffith Joyner and John Hanc (IDG Books Worldwide, Inc.)

Why You May Want to Try Walk-Run

By sprinkling running intervals throughout your walking workout, you can spike up exercise intensity and burn more calories. But I don't want you to come away with the impression that walking is a second-class activity. On the contrary, walking at any speed can help you drop body fat and boost your cardiovascular fitness. These results have been proven by numerous research studies, most notably a 1990 study done at the Cooper Institute for Aerobic Research in Dallas. Even lifestyle walkers who walked less than 3 miles an hour enjoyed significant health benefits as long as they walked long enough and often enough.

For those who use running as their primary form of exercise, injury is practically unavoidable. Walkers, no matter what their speed, land with 1 to 1.5 times the force of their body weight per step, while runners impact with 3 to 4 times their body weight. That extra impact can really take its toll on your body if all you do is run.

If you're interested in building speed and burning maximum calories, you may want to at least try a walk-run workout once in a while. Picking up the pace for short running intervals makes you work harder without overtaxing you or your joints for long periods of time. It's just another way to get more bang for your fitness buck. For those who want to run without blowing out their knees, ankles, hips, or lower back, walk-run is the perfect hybrid workout and a great way to train.

If, however, even short jogging stints make your knees ache, stick with pure walking. You can substitute high-energy walking intervals for the running intervals and get a similar workout.

How Much Is Enough?

Do up to three walk-run workouts a week. Walk-run is ideal for the days you want to push yourself a bit harder. If you are a runner, consider doing 1 to 2 days of walk-run to give your body a break from the daily pounding. But this message bears repeating: You never have to try walk-run if running even a step doesn't suit your body or your personality. It is simply another way to increase exercise intensity. If walk-run appeals to you, go for it. If it doesn't, don't feel as if you are settling for second best.

The amount of running that you insert into your program is another matter to consider. You may want to start out with just a few 1-minute intervals to see how it feels and gradually increase over time until you are running about half the time. I encourage you to play with the amounts of running you do. There is no set formula. Add in your running time slowly and carefully so that you can easily determine the amount of running your body is equipped to handle without breaking down.

Determining intensity

Base both your walking and running intensity on your ability, your current fitness level, and how you feel during each workout. Because walk-run is a form of interval training — alternating fast-paced intervals with slower-paced intervals — your intensity varies within each workout.

Start your walk-run workouts with 5 to 10 minutes of an easy walking warm-up followed by 20 to 45 minutes of moderate-to-challenging walk-run. Finish with a cool-down for 5 to 10 minutes at an easy walking pace. Check out the sample walk-run routines in this chapter for some typical ways to structure a walk-run workout.

When you first try walk-run, I recommend starting out with all moderate-intensity intervals (both walking and running) and then seeing how you hold up from there. In general, start out by running roughly 10 percent of your total workout time and than gradually increase the amount of running you do until you are running about half of the time. After you get the hang of walk-run, you can experiment with more challenging walking and running intervals.

Focusing on Form

During each walk-run workout, you will probably spend some time walking at several different levels although for the most part, you'll fitness walk. Refer to Chapters 7, 8, and 9 for a review on walking form at various levels.

Running is a different activity entirely from walking. During walking, you always have one foot in contact with the ground, whereas during running, you are airborne for a brief moment. When you run, you use more of your body, and you use your body differently. Even so, as you can see in the posture checklist in this section, running posture (shown in Figure 10-1) bears some similarities to walking posture.

Checking your running posture

- ✔ **Head:** Keep your head up and centered between your shoulders. Keep your chin up and focus your eyes straight ahead. Your head and neck should "float" above your shoulders in a relaxed, easy manner.
- ✔ **Shoulders:** Keep them back and down. Don't allow them to round forward or creep up toward your ears.
- ✔ **Chest:** Run tall. Keep your chest lifted naturally and don't twist from side to side as you run.

✔ **Arms:** Your arms should be bent to slightly less than 90 degrees. Swing them back and forth — not side to side — and keep them close to your body. At the top of your arm swing, your elbow is level with your breastbone; at the bottom of your swing, your hand brushes your hip.

✔ **Hands:** Keep them loosely cupped as if you are holding a butterfly in your hand that you don't want to let escape but that you don't want to crush either.

✔ **Abdominals:** Pull your belly button gently in toward your spine and tuck your pelvis forward ever so slightly so that you feel tall, stable, and upright. This position also protects your lower back.

✔ **Hips:** Power your movements from your hips rather than your thighs, but keep your hips loose and natural. Align them with your shoulders so that you can power your stride with maximum energy. Your hips should move forward and back rather than from side to side.

✔ **Thighs:** Lift your knees and extend your back leg to slightly lengthen your stride.

✔ **Feet:** Land firmly on your heel and roll smoothly to push off with your toes. Think of planting your heel and then "pushing the ground away from you" as you roll through your foot.

✔ **Breathing and heart rate:** Strive to keep your breathing deep but steady. Time your breathing so that it is in rhythm with your footfall.

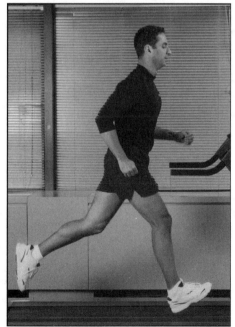

Figure 10-1: Here's a demonstration of good running posture.

Transition form

Be conscious of form lapses during transitions between walking and running. You have the greatest tendency to fall apart during these periods. Some common mistakes that occur during walk-to-run and run-to-walk transitions include the following:

- ✔ Your upper body posture falls apart. Your shoulders round forward, and your chest draws inward.

- ✔ Your arms begin to swing across your body, and your shoulders creep up toward your ears.

- ✔ Your lower back arches, and your abs go slack. As a result, you may also lock your knees for several transition strides.

- ✔ You fall forward, moving up onto your toes and limiting heel contact with the ground.

When transitioning between different gaits, keep these form mistakes in mind and try to avoid them. Maintaining proper form is probably hardest to do after a particularly challenging interval. If you've been giving it your all and you're ready to stop, good posture is probably not the first thing on your mind. Ease up and slow down somewhat gradually instead of immediately pouring on the gas or slamming on the breaks — take a few strides to complete each transition.

Developing a Walk-Run Routine

The walk-run routines in this section are designed to gradually increase the amount of time you spend running, your total workout time, your workout intensity, and the number of calories you burn per workout. Start out with the first set of beginner routines; they introduce a small amount of running so that you can see how your body reacts to this activity.

The first beginner routine (see Table 10-1), for instance, involves only 3 minutes of running. That may not sound like a lot, but it is. You may feel sore for a few days after your first walk-run workout, and if you do, that's normal. But if you feel aches and pains in your joints, running isn't for you, so consider using other ways of pumping up your walking routine.

The second set of routines, for intermediates (see Table 10-2), increases both the total amount of running and overall workout intensity. Stick with the beginner routines for a month or so and then give the intermediate routines a try. The third set of routines (see Table 10-3) is very advanced because of the amount of running you do and the high level of intensity you must maintain

throughout. You can give them a try after a month or so of doing the intermediate routines at least once a week. But you don't have to progress beyond
the beginner level if you don't want to.

The gradual approach to adding running to your workout helps you intensify
your fitness routine without inviting injury. A gradual increase in total
running mileage and running intensity is important because running can be
so hard on your body. Runners and those who walk-run can get injured when
they try to do too much too soon.

Table 10-1	Beginning Walk-Run Routines	
Routine 1	*Routine 2*	*Routine 3*
Walk 5 minutes EASY	Walk 5 minutes EASY	Walk 5 minutes EASY
Walk 5 minutes MODERATE	Walk 5 minutes MODERATE	Walk 5 minutes MODERATE
Run 1 minute EASY	Run 2 minutes EASY	Run 3 minutes EASY
Walk 5 minutes MODERATE	Walk 5 minutes MODERATE	Walk 5 minutes MODERATE
Run 1 minute EASY	Run 2 minutes EASY	Run 3 minutes EASY
Walk 5 minutes MODERATE	Walk 5 minutes MODERATE	Walk 5 minutes MODERATE
Run 1 minute EASY	Run 2 minutes EASY	Run 3 minutes EASY
Walk 3 minutes MODERATE	Walk 3 minutes MODERATE	Walk 3 minutes MODERATE
Walk 3 minutes EASY	Walk 3 minutes EASY	Walk 3 minutes EASY
Total walk time: 26 minutes	Total walk time: 26 minutes	Total walk time: 26 minutes
Total run time: 3 minutes	Total run time: 6 minutes	Total run time: 9 minutes
Total workout time: 29 minutes	Total workout time: 32 minutes	Total workout time: 35 minutes
Estimated calorie burn: 175	Estimated calorie burn: 205	Estimated calorie burn: 240

Table 10-2	Intermediate Walk-Run Routines	
Routine 1	*Routine 2*	*Routine 3*
Walk 5 minutes EASY	Walk 5 minutes EASY	Walk 5 minutes EASY
Walk 3 minutes MODERATE	Walk 3 minutes CHALLENGING	Walk 4 minutes CHALLENGING
Run 3 minutes EASY	Run 3 minutes MODERATE	Run 4 minutes MODERATE
Walk 3 minutes MODERATE	Walk 3 minutes CHALLENGING	Walk 4 minutes CHALLENGING
Run 3 minutes EASY	Run 3 minutes MODERATE	Run 4 minutes MODERATE
Walk 3 minutes MODERATE	Walk 3 minutes CHALLENGING	Walk 5 minutes CHALLENGING
Run 3 minutes EASY	Run 3 minutes MODERATE	Run 4 minutes MODERATE
Walk 3 minutes MODERATE	Walk 3 minutes MODERATE	Walk 3 minutes MODERATE
Run 3 minutes EASY	Run 3 minutes EASY	Run 3 minutes EASY
Walk 3 minutes MODERATE	Walk 3 minutes MODERATE	Walk 3 minutes MODERATE
Walk 3 minutes EASY	Walk 3 minutes EASY	Walk 3 minutes EASY
Total walk time: 23 minutes	Total walk time: 23 minutes	Total walk time: 27 minutes
Total run time: 12 minutes	Total run time: 12 minutes	Total run time: 15 minutes
Total workout time: 35 minutes	Total workout time: 35 minutes	Total workout time: 42 minutes
Estimated calorie burn: 255	Estimated calorie burn: 290	Estimated calorie burn: 361

Table 10-3	Advanced Walk-Run Routines	
Routine 1	*Routine 2*	*Routine 3*
Walk 5 minutes EASY	Walk 5 minutes EASY	Walk 5 minutes EASY
Walk 3 minutes MODERATE	Walk 3 minutes MODERATE	Walk 4 minutes CHALLENGING
Run 3 minutes MODERATE	Run 4 minutes MODERATE	Run 4 minutes CHALLENGING
Walk 3 minutes CHALLENGING	Walk 4 minutes CHALLENGING	Walk 4 minutes CHALLENGING
Run 3 minutes MODERATE	Run 4 minutes MODERATE	Run 4 minutes CHALLENGING
Walk 3 minutes CHALLENGING	Walk 4 minutes CHALLENGING	Walk 5 minutes CHALLENGING
Run 3 minutes MODERATE	Run 4 minutes MODERATE	Run 4 minutes CHALLENGING
Walk 3 minutes CHALLENGING	Walk 4 minutes CHALLENGING	Walk 3 minutes CHALLENGING
Run 3 minutes MODERATE	Run 4 minutes MODERATE	Run 3 minutes CHALLENGING
Walk 3 minutes CHALLENGING	Walk 4 minutes CHALLENGING	Walk 3 minutes CHALLENGING
Walk 3 minutes EASY	Walk 3 minutes EASY	Walk 3 minutes EASY
Total walk time: 23 minutes	Total walk time: 27 minutes	Total walk time: 27 minutes
Total run time: 12 minutes	Total run time: 16 minutes	Total run time: 15 minutes
Total workout time: 35 minutes	Total workout time: 43 minutes	Total workout time: 42 minutes
Estimated calorie burn: 302	Estimated calorie burn: 386	Estimated calorie burn: 409

The sample workouts in this section refer to the terms "easy," "moderate," and "challenging" to help define the intensity of your workouts. Here is a detailed explanation of what these terms mean.

Easy

Easy intensity refers to a comfortable pace that you can keep up for quite a while whether you're walking or running. Here's how to tell whether you're working at an easy intensity:

- ✔ Your target heart rate is 50 to 60 percent of your age-predicted maximum heart rate. See Chapter 5 for information on how to calculate both your maximum and target heart rates.

- ✔ Your rating of perceived exertion (RPE) is between 4 and 6. Check out Chapter 5 for a complete explanation of RPE and how to determine yours.

- ✔ Your breathing is steady, and you can carry on a normal but breathy conversation.

- ✔ Most people are at an easy intensity level when they are walking at 2.5 to 3.5 miles per hour. Typically, you are lifestyle walking at this level of intensity.

- ✔ Most people are at an easy intensity when they are running at about 4 to 5.5 miles per hour. Typically, you are at a lope or a relaxed jog at this level of intensity.

Moderate

At a moderate intensity, you are pushing but still maintaining a comfortable walking or running speed. Here's how to tell whether you're working at a moderate intensity:

- ✔ Your target heart rate is 60 to 75 percent of your age-predicted maximum heart rate. See Chapter 5 for information on how to calculate both your maximum and target heart rates.

- ✔ Your rating of perceived exertion (RPE) is between 6 and 8. Check out Chapter 5 for a complete explanation of RPE and how to determine yours.

- ✔ Your breathing is deep but regular. You can still carry on a conversation but perhaps not as well as when you move at an easy pace.

- ✔ Most people are at a moderate intensity level when they are walking at 3.5 to 4.5 miles per hour. Typically, you are fitness walking at this level of intensity.

- ✔ Most people are at a moderate intensity when they are running at about 5.5 to 6.5 miles per hour. Typically, you are at a fast but comfortable jog or run at this level of intensity.

Challenging

Now you're working hard! Here's how to tell whether you're working at a challenging intensity:

- Your target heart rate is 75 to 95 percent of your age-predicted maximum heart rate. See Chapter 5 for information on how to calculate both your maximum and target heart rates.

- Your rating of perceived exertion (RPE) is between 8 and 10. Check out Chapter 5 for a complete explanation of RPE and how to determine yours.

- Your breathing is deep and very loud. You can still carry on snatches of conversation, although talking is still somewhat difficult. You feel your blood pumping, your heart pounding, and your muscles working at near max.

- Most people are at a challenging intensity level when they are walking 4.5 to 6.0 miles per hour. Typically, you are high-energy walking at this level of intensity.

- Most people are at a challenging intensity when they are running at about 6.5 to 8.0 miles per hour. Typically, you are running at a fast clip. Although you don't have to, you can do a near all-out sprint.

Calorie Counter

Use Table 10-4 to determine how many calories you burn for each minute of running you do. Simply look up how many calories you burn per minute based upon your body weight and multiply it by the number of minutes you run. You can estimate your total walk-run calorie burn by combining the total time you walk with the total amount of time you run. You can find calorie counts for each of the different levels of walking in Chapters 7 through 9.

Table 10-4	Calories Burned during Running		
Body Weight (In Pounds)	Easy Running	Moderate Running	Challenging Running
	Estimated Calorie Burn at Average Speed 5.0 mph	Estimated Calorie Burn at Average Speed 6.0 mph	Estimated Calorie Burn at Average Speed 7.0 mph
115 to 125	8.5 calories/minute	10 calories/minute	11.5 calories/minute
130 to 140	9.5 calories/minute	11 calories/minute	13 calories/minute
145 to 155	10.5 calories/minute	12.5 calories/minute	14 calories/minute
160 to 170	11.5 calories/minute	14 calories/minute	15.5 calories/minute
175 to 185	13 calories/minute	15 calories/minute	17 calories/minute
190 to 200	14 calories/minute	16 calories/minute	18.5 calories/minute
205 to 215	15 calories/minute	17 calories/minute	20 calories/minute
220 to 230	16 calories/minute	18.5 calories/minute	21 calories/minute
235 to 245	17 calories/minute	20 calories/minute	23 calories/minute

Minding Your Pace

In this chapter, I talk a lot about how fast you walk or run. Do you want to determine your exact pace or speed? Grab your sports watch or stopwatch and find a quarter-mile track at your local high school or university. Time a quarter mile at easy, moderate, and challenging walking paces and at easy, moderate, and challenging running paces. Then multiply each of those quarter-mile times by 4 to come up with your per-mile time or pace. *Pace* refers to how many minutes it takes to cover 1 mile, whereas *speed* is measured in miles per hour or the amount of distance you cover in 1 hour. Refer to the pace/speed conversion chart in Table 10-5 to see how a specific pace and speed relate to one another.

If you do all six time trials on the same day, that's six laps around the track in total — quite a workout. But you don't have to do them all in one session if you don't want to. Be sure to warm up for 5 minutes or so before attempting any moderate or challenging time trials. Cool down for 5 minutes or so, too.

Table 10-5	Pace/Speed Conversion Chart
Walking	
Pace (Minutes per Mile)	*Speed (Miles per Hour)*
30.0	2.0
24.0	2.5
20.0	3.0
17.1	3.5
Walking or Running	
Pace (Minutes per Mile)	*Speed (Miles per Hour)*
15	4.0
13.3	4.5
12.0	5.0
10.9	5.5
Running	
Pace (Minutes per Mile)	*Speed (Miles per Hour)*
10.0	6.0
9.2	6.5
8.5	7.0
8.0	7.5
7.5	8.0
7.0	8.5
6.6	9.0
6.3	9.5
6.0	10.0

Part III
Beyond the Basics

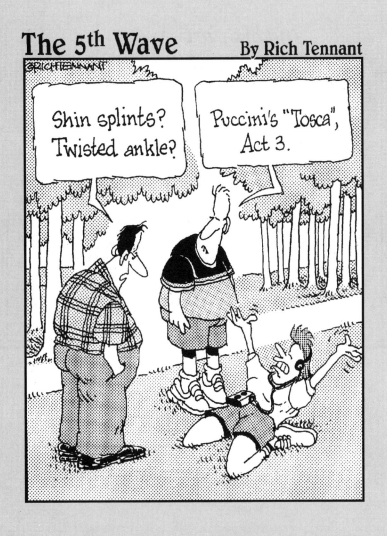

In this part . . .

This section explains how to get the biggest bang for your walking — and exercise — buck. Chapter 11 describes the best strength training exercises for walkers, followed by Chapter 12, which describes the best stretches for walkers. Chapter 13 introduces you to advanced training techniques like intervals and tempos. If you have a special need to consider when you walk, flip to Chapter 14. This chapter contains information on how to modify your walking program if you're pregnant or a little older, or if you consider yourself extremely out of shape. Though walkers are typically blessed with a low injury rate, Chapter 15 tells you how to avoid injuring yourself and how to deal with aches and pains as they come up. Chapter 16 is devoted to walking workouts on the tread-mill. I give you pointers on how to buy a treadmill, how to use one, and how to take the boredom out of walking to nowhere. Chapter 17 covers walking through the woods, around the mall, along the beach, and in your swimming pool.

Chapter 11

Strength Training Exercises for Walkers

. . . .

In This Chapter

▶ Understanding why walkers need to weight train

▶ Muscling your way through the terminology

▶ Getting the right equipment

▶ Exercising with weights

. . . .

You've already committed or are at least thinking about committing a certain amount of time and energy to a walking program, so why should you add yet another activity to your exercise repertoire?

It's probably not good enough for me to say "because I say so" or "because it's good for you," so here's the real reason: A complete fitness routine contains three equally important elements: cardiovascular endurance (walking), flexibility (stretching, which I explain in Chapter 6), and strength (weight training). Each of these three fitness components complements and bolsters the others. If you're lacking in one area, you won't reap the full benefits of the others.

I cover the who, what, where, when, why, and how of weight training in this chapter.

Four Reasons Walkers Should Weight Train

You only need to devote about 20 minutes, twice a week, to weight training, but that 40 minutes a week will pay you back in spades. Considering what it can do for you, the minimal commitment that weight training requires is definitely worth it. In case you're not convinced, here are four compelling reasons to work out with weights.

Weight training prevents injury

Although walking is low impact and safe, many walkers experience ankle, knee, hip, or lower back pain at some point in their career. Sometimes this pain is a result of walking, and sometimes it results from doing other forms of exercise. Injuries can also be the result of a traumatic event like a fall or the wrong step off a curb. Strong muscles support and protect your joints, thus lessening the chance of injury to these hot spots. Even if you do fall, the stronger your muscles are, the less damage you're likely to do. If you already have an injury, a combination of weight training and stretching can help it heal more quickly and may help alleviate chronic problems.

Weight training enhances performance

Strong leg and buttocks muscles lend your walking stride purpose and power. They make it easier to charge up hills and sprint toward home. Strong upper body muscles contribute to a more forceful arm swing. Strong middle body muscles help you maintain good walking posture. Good walking posture helps prevent fatigue and allows you to maintain deep, regular breathing. In short, strong muscles allow you to walk farther, faster, and longer.

Weight training helps prevent osteoporosis

Osteoporosis is a condition characterized by low bone density. It leads to brittle, weak, and porous bones that break easily and do not support your body properly. Older women in particular are susceptible to osteoporosis and osteoarthritis. In fact, the average woman loses about 1 percent of her overall bone density each year after the age of 35.

If you break or fracture an already weakened bone, it may not heal properly for weeks or even months. Until recently, we accepted this as an inevitable fact of aging. There is now evidence that bone loss can be prevented or slowed down through a combination of diet and exercise. Many respected professional organizations, including the American College of Sports Medicine, now recommend a combination of land-based aerobic exercise; a calcium-, vitamin D-, and protein-rich diet; and regular weight training (including weight-bearing activity) as the best defense against osteoporosis for both women and men.

A regular walking routine covers the land-based activity part of the equation. Walking provides enough stimulation to help preserve bone density in the bones of your lower body. But walking alone is not enough to prevent bone density loss entirely.

Osteoporosis is joint specific. The bones you "stress" are the bones that harden. Bones that receive no stimuli are still in danger of losing valuable calcium and other minerals. That's where weight training comes in.

Weight training causes the muscles you train to pull on your bones. This places stress on the joints and bones that the muscles attach to and signals them to stimulate and preserve bone material. For example, when you do a front shoulder raise (described later in this chapter), the shoulder muscles pull on the humerous and scapula bones that form your shoulder joint. Because weight training is site specific, you can focus on individual areas of your body, including the hips, thighs, and shoulders — three of the most common sites of fractures in older individuals.

Weight training helps you lose weight and maintain weight loss

Here's the theory: Muscle tissue requires more energy to maintain than fat tissue, so the more muscle you pack on your body, the more calories you burn throughout the day, even while at rest. For every 1 pound of muscle you gain, you burn an extra 150 calories a day. Over the course of a year, this can add up to a weight loss of 10 pounds. To look at it another way, it can prevent you from *gaining* 10 pounds a year. Of course, the amount of weight you lose (or don't gain) depends upon how much you eat, how many additional calories you burn, and your individual metabolism.

Many people avoid weight lifting because they think that it will cause them to "bulk up" or at least prevent them from losing weight. Actually, once you start lifting weights, the needle on the bathroom scale may not creep downward as quickly as you'd like. But if you take out a tape measure, you will probably find that you are losing inches. How is this possible? Muscle is denser than fat, so it takes up less room. The more muscular you are, the tighter, firmer, and thinner you appear — even if you never lose a pound.

Bodybuilders and other athletes would be labeled as overweight only if you considered their scale weights. But no one would accuse skater Katerina Witt or professional basketball player Lisa Leslie of being too fat. Their weight is predominantly lean body mass, and their body composition — ratio of fat to muscle — is within a healthy range.

Getting a Grip on Muscle Lingo

Your body contains over 600 muscles. Fortunately, you need to be familiar with only about a dozen of them for our purposes. That's because a walker's weight training routine — like most other weight training routines — focuses only on larger, frequently used muscles collectively known as *the major muscle groups.*

Including at least one exercise for every major muscle group in your weight-training routine on a regular basis develops balanced muscle strength, helps prevent walking injuries, and enhances your walking performance.

As a walker, you may be surprised that you need to strengthen more than just your thighs. Walking involves virtually all your major muscle groups to a varying degree. Although your thighs and buttocks carry you forward, your abdominal and other torso muscles keep you upright, and your upper body muscles provide the force for your arm swing.

In the following sections, I provide a brief anatomy lesson about those major muscle groups and how each of them contributes to a successful walking program. I've always believed that the more you know about what you're doing, the more likely you are to do it correctly. I start with the larger muscles and work down to the smallest muscles within the context of the lower, upper, and middle sections of your body — which is exactly how a proper weight training routine should be organized.

Your lower body muscles

The largest muscles in your body are all located south of your waistline. These are obviously the muscles that are responsible for the bulk of the work when you walk. It's important to put them through a regular regimen of strength training to make you a stronger walker and to prevent hip, knee, and ankle problems.

- **Buttocks:** I probably don't have to tell you that your buttocks, or *gluteus maximus,* comprise the largest muscle in your entire body. It spans the entire width of your rear and is responsible for lifting your leg upward to take a stride. The "glutes" come into play even more when you walk fast or walk up hills. Both activities require a higher leg lift.

- **Thighs:** The muscles in the front of your thigh are called the *quadriceps,* or "quads"; the muscles in the back of your thighs are called the *hamstrings,* or "hams." Together they are responsible for straightening and bending your knee, a function that's obviously needed in walking. (Your hamstrings also help lower your leg as you complete a stride.) Both of these muscle groups must be strong and in balance to prevent knee problems.

✔ **Lower legs:** The *gastrocnemius* and the *soleus* are the two largest muscles in the back of your lower leg. Together they are known as the calf muscles and power your toe lift and foot plant. Because they are among the most often used muscle groups in your body, they are specially geared toward fatigue resistance. Thus, strong calves play a key role in long-term endurance.

Your upper body muscles

Why should walkers even bother thinking about their upper body muscles? Because your arm swing provides a lot of the power and rhythm involved in walking. Working your upper body muscles so that they are strong and in shape will undoubtedly make you a better walker.

✔ **Upper back:** There are several large muscles in your upper back; the largest is named the *latissimus dorsi,* or "lats" for short. Other upper back muscles include the rhomboids and the trapezius. Your upper back muscles are an important part of both good posture and proper arm swing. Without good upper back strength, you will round forward. This posture can lead to premature fatigue and breathing difficulties.

✔ **Chest:** Otherwise known as your *pectorals,* your chest muscles extend the width of the front of your upper body from your armpit to just below the nipple line. They work in opposition to your upper back muscles to provide power for the forward part of your arm swing. They are also one of the keys to good, uplifted upper body posture.

✔ **Shoulders:** The *deltoids,* or "delts" for short, include the four muscles that form a muscular cap around the top of your arm. (The rotator cuff muscles lie underneath them.) Your delts assist in both the forward and backward portion of your arm swing. In terms of posture, their contribution cannot be understated.

Nothing looks worse or decreases your performance more than stooped and rounded shoulders. You'll notice that most of the exercise descriptions later in this chapter contain reminders to maintain good shoulder positioning.

✔ **Arms:** Are you getting the idea that most major muscle groups have cute little nicknames? Well, the biceps muscles located in the front of your upper arm and the triceps muscles located in the back of your upper arm are no exception: They're referred to as your "bis" and "tris," respectively. They help hold your arms in the proper bend position and contribute to the strength of your arm swing.

Your middle body muscles

The muscles of your middle body allow you to stand and walk with good posture. Strengthening these muscles should help you avoid lower back pain as well.

- ✔ **Abdominals:** Your "abs" are the most essential postural muscles in your body. They include all the muscles that wrap around your mid-torso to form a sort of anatomic support girdle. Without strong abs, you could not stand erect, let alone walk with the proper upright posture. Strong abs also protect against lower back fatigue and ultimately lower back pain and discomfort.

- ✔ **Erector spinae:** These muscles run in parallel tracks along either side of your spine. For simplicity's sake, the bottom half of these muscles are collectively referred to as the "lower back muscles." Along with the abs, they contribute to good walking posture and prevent low back exhaustion.

Weight Training Basics

Like anything else, weight training has some fundamental guidelines you need to know about. These rules go a long way toward making your weight training experience a sane and sensible one. I promise to keep these rules and regulations as simple as possible. If you are interested in learning about more advanced weight training techniques, I suggest that you pick up *Weight Training For Dummies* by Liz Neporent and Suzanne Schlosberg (IDG Books Worldwide, Inc.).

Actually weight training is synonymous with two other terms: *strength training* and *resistance training*. Strength training includes any exercise that is done specifically to strengthen muscles or improve local *muscular endurance* (the stamina of the individual muscle being worked.)

Exercises that build strength involve working a muscle against some type of resistance — hence the name resistance training — for a relatively short period of time. The weights you use for the exercises later in this chapter are one type of resistance. Other examples of things that can provide resistance include your body, gravity, soup cans, your cat, a lamp, this book — anything that a muscle must fight against in order to move. In order for a resistance to be effective, it must place the working muscle under more stress than it is typically used to. This extra work is what forces the muscles to adapt, build, strengthen, and grow.

Understanding training terminology

In general, you are using the correct amount of resistance if you can lift a weight 8 to 15 times in a row without stopping. If you can't lift it at least 8 times without struggling or breaking form, the resistance is too heavy. If you can lift it 15 times in a row without exerting much of an effort, it is probably too light.

Each complete rendition (one lift and one lower) of an exercise is called a *repetition* (or *rep*). One rep of a biceps curl, for example, involves bending your arm and then straightening it. One complete cycle of reps is known as a *set*. Fifteen reps of a biceps curl equal one set.

How many sets and reps of each exercise you should do depends upon your goals. If your goal is to build a moderate amount of strength, improve your health, prevent injuries, and enhance your walking performance, then doing one set of each exercise in this chapter at least twice a week is sufficient. If you have more high-minded athletic goals — such as competing in a race walking event or building and sculpting your body — you need to do 3 or more sets for each major muscle group, including your back, chest, shoulders, arms, abs, thighs, and buttocks. (For a more detailed description of the major muscle groups, refer to the "Getting a Grip on Muscle Lingo" section earlier in this chapter.)

For most recreational walkers, 2 to 3 weekly weight training workouts consisting of 1 to 3 sets of about 10 exercises using moderately heavy weights will suffice.

Don't weight train two days in a row. If you lift on Monday, for example, don't lift again until Wednesday. The reason? Weight training literally tears your muscles apart. Resting them for at least 48 hours between workouts allows them to repair and grow stronger. And without adequate rest, you increase the risk of injury.

Getting the essential equipment

In this section, I provide a list of essential weight training equipment. I tried to keep the amount of weight training equipment you'll need to a minimum. All told, a complete setup shouldn't cost more than $150. I also try to give as many exercise modifications as possible that require no equipment at all. The following sections detail the equipment you need to get started.

Aerobic step

Aerobic steps can be purchased at sporting good stores or even department stores. Besides being a handy, easily stored weight bench, you can use a step to do aerobic exercise on cross-training days when you don't walk. Prices range from $30 to $120.

The best steps consist of a rectangular *platform* and several sets of stackable *risers* that snap on underneath the platform to raise and lower the height of the step.

Look for a step that's made of unbreakable plastic. It should have some type of no-skid, rubberized material on the top of the platform to prevent it from getting slippery when wet. It should be long enough so that when you lie down, your entire body, from your head to your tailbone, fits on the platform; it's okay if your legs hang off. I recommend staying away from steps made of foam or Styrofoam because they are not as sturdy and tend to fall apart after a few months of regular use.

The brands I like the best are The Step and Reebok (ordering information is included in the appendix). You cannot go wrong with either of these.

Dumbbells

Dumbbells are short-handled metal bars with a "head" attached to each end. Heads are round or hexagonal or shaped like flat disks. They are either welded permanently to the ends of the bar or slide on and off so that you can adjust the weight of the bar. Screws, pins, or collars clamp weight plates onto the bar.

Because weight is weight, don't throw away big bucks purchasing shiny chrome "beauty" bells unless you want to make a statement. Cheap, gray, painted hexagonal dumbbells are just fine and run from 10 cents to 85 cents a pound depending on what part of the country you live in and where you buy them. You can probably hunt down a perfectly acceptable set of weights for just pennies at a garage sale. If you do buy them secondhand, make sure that the heads are securely attached to the bars, the paint isn't flaking, and, if they're adjustable, all the parts are included or replacement parts are easy to find.

I personally prefer solid weights to adjustable weights. The weight plates on most adjustable sets tend to wobble around. In the worst-case scenario, they can slide off and give you a memorable bruise on top of your foot. Trust me, I've been there. And when you're trying to bang through a training session, isn't it easier to simply pick up the correct weight as opposed to stopping, popping off the collars, setting up the new weight, and then redoing the collars?

Solid weights do cost you more because you need to buy several sets. It's highly unlikely that you'll use the same weight for every exercise. Despite the extra expense, I think you'll find the convenience of solid weights worth it in the long run.

If you don't want to make any financial commitment whatsoever to weight lifting, you can raid your kitchen cupboard for a no-cost dumbbell alternative. Soup cans and other canned products make fine dumbbells when you don't need a very heavy weight. (They also make a healthy post-workout snack if you lift the no-salt products.) Typically, cans weigh from 1 to 3 pounds. Just make sure that you use cans of equal weight and that you can grasp them firmly and comfortably. As you get stronger, you'll probably outgrow chicken-and-rice-sized resistance. At that point, you can use bleach bottles filled with water, dried beans, or sand. Again, just make sure that your homemade dumbbells are equal in weight and easy to grip.

Exercise mat

If you are so inclined, you can buy a special exercise mat for floor exercises and stretches. The extra padding it provides will save your joints and make the exercises more comfortable. For a decent foldable, washable exercise mat, expect to pay anywhere from $30 to $100.

Everlast and Airex are two brands of exercise mats that I like. Of course, a thick blanket or beach towel is an acceptable substitute.

Chair

Some of the exercise options that I provide call for a sturdy chair to hold on to for support and balance.

Don't buy any special type of chair for exercise purposes. Use a desk or kitchen chair that does not have rollers and will not slide around when you lean some of your weight against it. Bed posts, pillars, and walls are suitable substitutes as well.

The Walker's Weight Training Routine

In this section, I provide ten strength training exercises specifically geared toward the muscles walkers use and the way they use them. At the beginning of each exercise, I describe the purpose of the exercise and tell you about the muscles being worked. I also provide plenty of technique tips and modifications, so be sure to read those carefully.

These are by no means the only acceptable exercises. You have literally hundreds of exercise to choose from. If you decide that you like training with weights, look for more detailed information on the topic.

Your local bookstore has dozens of related weight training titles. Monthly magazines such as *Shape, Fitness,* and *Men's Health* contain creative and sensible weight workouts in each issue.

The exercises in this chapter form a routine. Do them in the order listed, working your larger muscles first and then your smaller ones. This is the safest, not to mention the most effective, way to get the job done. Start with one set of 8 to 15 repetitions each. As you get stronger, you can increase the weight you use and/or increase the number of sets you do of each exercise to three if you want to up the intensity. After you are familiar with the routine, you should be able to complete it in no more than 20 minutes. I recommend doing two to three weight workouts a week, with at least one day of rest in between. Read the sidebar "The golden rules of weight training," later in this chapter, for universal training tips.

One last thing before you jump into those exercises: If you have never picked up a weight or haven't lifted in a while, be prepared to be sore for a few days afterward. This feeling is part of the normal adaptation process that your body goes through when it is learning a new skill. You can minimize this soreness by starting with light weights and taking plenty of rest between sets. A little achiness is almost impossible to avoid for a day or two after your first couple of lifts. However, if you are so sore that you can't stand up straight without help or lift your cereal spoon to your mouth without screaming in agony, you've probably overdone it.

Lunge

Purpose: This exercise is ideal for walkers because it mimics a walking stride. It strengthens the buttocks, hips, thighs, and lower leg.

Knees, lower back

Setup: Stand tall with your feet placed as wide as your hips, your slightly bent arms at your sides, and your hands in loose fists, as shown in Figure 11-1a.

Pull your abdominals gently inward and keep your shoulders back.

Movement: Leading with your heel, step your right leg a stride's length forward. As your heel makes contact with the floor, bend both knees so that your right thigh is parallel to the floor and your left thigh is perpendicular to it (see Figure 11-1b). Press through the ball of the foot to stand back up. Repeat, leading with your left leg. Alternate sides until you have completed all reps.

Do's and Don'ts:

✔ As you do the exercise, do imagine you're stepping over a crack on the sidewalk.

✔ Do swing your opposite arm forward as you step to give the movement power and balance.

✔ Do allow your back heel to lift off the floor as you bend your knees.

✔ Don't allow your upper body to round or fall forward or your front knee to travel forward of your toes.

Modifications:

✔ **Balance lunge:** If you have trouble maintaining balance, place a sturdy chair to one side of you and hold onto it.

✔ **Weighted lunge:** Hold a dumbbell in each hand to add resistance to this exercise. In this version, your arms should remain at your sides throughout.

✔ **Split lunge or split squat:** Begin with your legs already straddled a stride length's distance apart. Bend your knees so that the lowered position looks like the movement of the basic lunge.

✔ **Step up:** If you hike or walk a lot of hills, try this version: Place one to three sets of risers underneath your step platform and place the step a stride's length in front of you. As you lunge forward, step your entire foot onto the platform of the step.

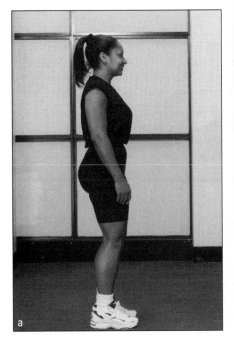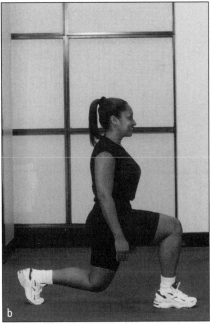

Figure 11-1:
Keep your shoulders back when performing lunges.

Calf raise

Purpose: This exercise strengthens and stretches your calf muscles, which, along with your other lower leg muscles, are needed for a firm foot plant and overall stamina.

Setup: Place your step against a wall and stand on the step so that your heels are hanging off the edge. You can place your hands against the wall for balance.

Stand tall with your abdominals gently pulled inward and your straightened legs hip-width apart.

Movement: Raise up on your tiptoes as high as you can (see Figure 11-2a). Hold a moment and slowly lower so that your heels dip slightly below the platform and you feel a stretch through your calves (see Figure 11-2b).

Do's:

- Do imagine that you are trying to peek over the top of a fence.
- Do keep your legs straight.

Modifications:

- **One-legger:** To isolate one leg at a time, bend your left leg and wrap your foot behind your right ankle so that you are balanced on your right foot. Perform the exercise with your right leg and then repeat with your left leg. You can hold a dumbbell in your opposite hand to make this version more challenging.

- **Pulses:** For a greater challenge, stay up on your tiptoes and do 10 small, short reps before lowering your heels.

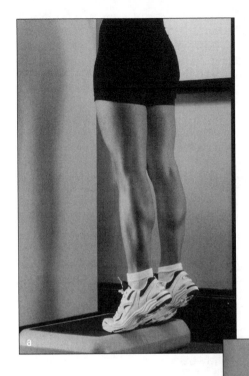

Figure 11-2:
This exercise strengthens your calf muscles.

Pullover

Purpose: The pullover improves your walking posture by strengthening the upper back, chest, shoulders, and arm muscles.

Shoulders

Setup: Hold a single dumbbell with both hands and lie on a bench with your knees bent and your feet flat on the bench. Raise your arms directly over your shoulders. Turn your palms up so that one end of the dumbbell is resting in the gap between your palms and the other end is hanging straight down over your chest, as shown in Figure 11-3a.

Pull your abdominals in, but make sure that your back is relaxed and arched naturally.

Movement: Lower the dumbbell behind you until the bottom head of it is level with the back of your head (see Figure 11-3b). Restraighten your arms.

Do's and Don'ts:

✔ Do imagine that you are raising and lowering an ax to chop wood.

✔ Do keep your elbows slightly bent.

✔ Don't arch your lower back as you lower the dumbbell.

✔ Don't lower the dumbbell too far.

Modifications:

✔ **Floor pullover:** Lie on the floor and do the exercise. Doing so restricts your shoulder movement.

✔ **Double pullover:** If one arm is obviously stronger than the other, try this version: Hold a dumbbell in each hand and perform the exercise.

✔ **Using a step and risers:** As with most exercises that call for you to use a bench, it's okay to substitute an aerobic step platform and one to three sets of risers under the platform.

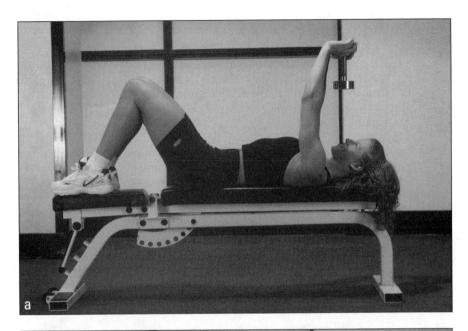

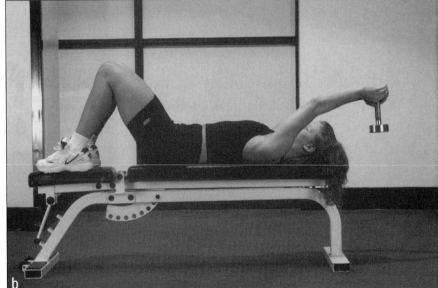

Figure 11-3:
You can see
how the
pullover
gets its
name.

Push-ups

Purpose: Strong chest muscles are an important part of good walking posture; triceps muscles contribute to a powerful arm swing. This exercise focuses on both of those muscle groups.

Shoulders, lower back

Setup: Lie on your stomach with your legs out straight. Bend your elbows and place your palms on the floor a bit to the side and in front of your shoulders. Straighten your arms and lift your body so that you're balanced on your palms and toes, as shown in Figure 11-4a.

Tuck your chin in a few inches toward your chest so that your forehead faces the floor. Tighten your abdominal muscles.

Movement: Bend your elbows and lower your entire body at once. Instead of trying to touch your chest to the floor, lower yourself only until your upper arms are parallel to the floor (see Figure 11-4b). Push yourself back up.

Do's and Don'ts:

- ✔ Do imagine that your upper and middle body are one unit and *must* move together in one straight line.

- ✔ Don't allow your back to sag.

- ✔ Don't completely lock your elbows at the top of the movement.

- ✔ Don't allow your head to dip forward of your shoulders.

- ✔ Don't lower yourself too far. Doing so can lead to shoulder and neck pain.

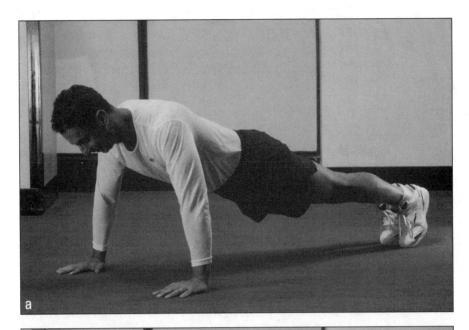

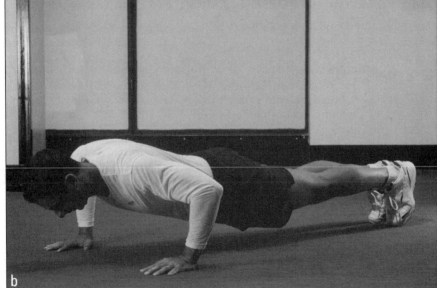

Figure 11-4: Push-ups can improve your posture and arm swing.

Front shoulder raise

Purpose: If you want to work your shoulders for a stronger arm pump, try this exercise.

Shoulders, rotator cuff

Setup: Stand tall with your feet hip-width apart. Hold a dumbbell in each hand. Place your arms in front of your thighs with your palms inward and the dumbbells resting against your thighs (see Figure 11-5a).

Pull your abs gently inward and keep your shoulders back.

Movement: Raise your right arm up until the dumbbell is level with your shoulder and slowly lower, as shown in Figure 11-5b. Repeat with your left arm. Alternate until you complete all reps.

Do's and Don'ts:

✔ Do imagine that you are raising a glass to toast a walk well done!

✔ Don't lift the dumbbell any higher than shoulder height.

✔ Don't arch your lower back or swing your body as you lift and lower the weight.

Modifications:

✔ **Palms up front raise:** If this move bothers your shoulders, do it with your palms turned upward.

✔ **Salutes:** If you have no shoulder or rotator cuff problems and want more of a challenge, try this: Start with your hands at your sides, palms inward. As you lift the weight, move your arm inward so that it is level with your opposite eye. Retrace your path to lower.

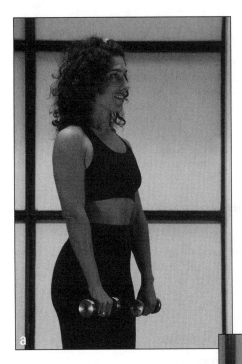

Figure 11-5:
The front shoulder raise can give you a stronger arm pump.

Back shoulder fly

Purpose: Because proper posture is such an important aspect of correct walking form, I include this exercise. It strengthens the upper back and shoulders and promotes postural awareness.

Shoulders, neck

Setup: Hold a dumbbell in each hand and stand with your feet hip-width apart. Bend your knees a few inches and lean forward from your hips. (See Figure 11-6a.)

Keep your abdominals pulled inward and your lower back straight. Let your arms hang straight down so that your palms are facing each other.

Movement: Bend your elbows and lift your arms up and out to the side until your elbows are level with your shoulder, as shown in Figure 11-6b. Slowly retrace your arclike path back to the start.

Do's and Don'ts:

- ✔ Do imagine that you are scooping up a big pile of clothes.
- ✔ Do keep your back flat throughout.
- ✔ Do keep your elbows slightly bent as you do this exercise.
- ✔ Don't allow your head to dip forward of your shoulders or your back to round.

Modifications:

- ✔ **Incline back shoulder fly:** If this exercise gives you a pain in the neck, incline one end of your step platform by using three risers. Lie face down on it with your head at the upper end and your legs kicked back behind you. Place a towel over the upper end of the platform and rest your chin on the towel so that your neck is relaxed.
- ✔ **Palms back shoulder fly:** For a different challenge, do this exercise with your palms facing backward.

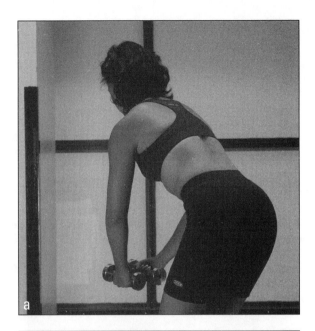

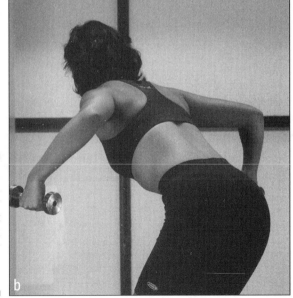

Figure 11-6:
Try the back shoulder fly if you want to work on your walking posture.

Biceps curl

Purpose: This exercise strengthens the biceps muscles, which are located in the front of the upper arm, and helps power your arm swing.

Elbows

Setup: Stand tall with your feet hip-width apart. Hold a dumbbell in each hand with your arms at your sides, palms facing inward (see Figure 11-7a).

Pull your abdominals gently inward and keep your shoulders back.

Movement: Bend your right arm and lift the weight until the dumbbell is at shoulder level, as shown in Figure 11-7b. Lower and repeat with the left arm. Repeat until you have completed all reps.

Do's and Don'ts:

✔ Do imagine that your arm is a nutcracker and you are trying to crack a large nut held in the well of your arm in front of your elbow.

✔ Do keep your knees slightly bent to protect your lower back.

✔ Do keep your elbows parallel to the sides of your body.

✔ Don't arch your back or swing as you lift and lower the weights.

Modifications:

✔ **Biceps curl with a twist:** For more of a challenge, start with your palms facing inward and, as you lift the weight, twist your hand around to the palms inward position. Retrace the path back to the start.

✔ **Hammer curl:** To place emphasis on the wrist muscles, start with your hands palms inward and maintain this position as you lift and lower the weights.

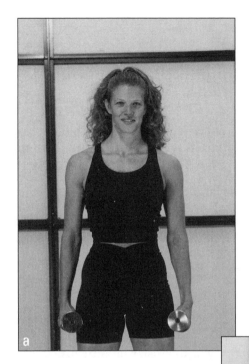

Figure 11-7:
Do the
biceps curl
to tone
your biceps
muscles.

Kickbacks

Purpose: This exercise strengthens the triceps muscles, which are located in the back of the upper arm and help power your arm swing.

Elbows

Setup: Hold a dumbbell in your right hand and stand with your feet hip-width apart. Bend your knees a few inches and lean forward from your hips. (See Figure 11-8a.)

Keep your abdominals pulled inward and your lower back straight. Place your left hand across your thighs for support. Bend your right arm and hold it up so that your upper arm is alongside your waist and your forearm is perpendicular to the floor.

Movement: Extend your right arm straight out behind you, as shown in Figure 11-8b. Return to the start. Complete all reps with your right arm and then do the same with your left arm.

Do's and Don'ts:

- ✔ Do imagine that you are trying to brush some crumbs off the side of your hip.
- ✔ Do keep your abdominals pulled in and your back straight.
- ✔ Do keep your shoulder still and move only from your elbow.
- ✔ Don't fully lock your elbow when you straighten your arm.

Modifications:

- ✔ **Double kickback:** For more of a challenge, work both arms at the same time.
- ✔ **Limited range kickback:** If the basic version bothers your elbow, straighten your arm only halfway or to a pain-free range of motion.

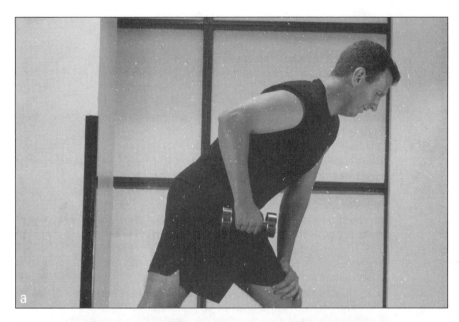

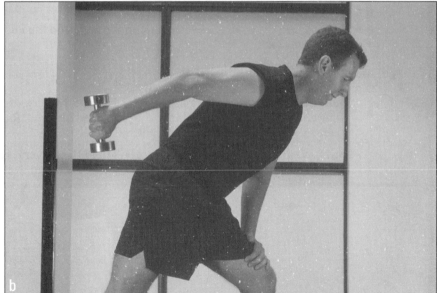

Figure 11-8:
Make kick-
backs a part
of your
routine.

Opposite extensions

Purpose: This exercise keeps your lower back strong and flexible.

Lower back

Setup: Lie on your stomach with your arms and legs outstretched (see Figure 11-9a).

Gently pull your abdominals inward and place your forehead on the floor so that your neck aligns with the rest of your spine.

Movement: Lift your right arm and left leg a few inches off the floor. Hold a moment, slowly lower, and then repeat the movement using your left arm and right leg (see Figure 11-9b). Alternate until you have completed all reps.

Do's:

- ✔ Do imagine that you are trying to reach something with your raised hand and toe that is just out of your reach.
- ✔ Do try to stretch out longer instead of raising your arm and leg higher.
- ✔ Do maintain the space between your abdominals and the floor to protect your lower back.

Modifications:

- ✔ **Modified back raise:** If the basic version bothers your lower back, fold your arms in front of you and rest your forehead on them. Raise your right leg up and hold and then repeat with your left leg.
- ✔ **Swimming:** For more of a challenge, don't hold the movement at the top. Instead, alternate quickly, as if you were moving through water.

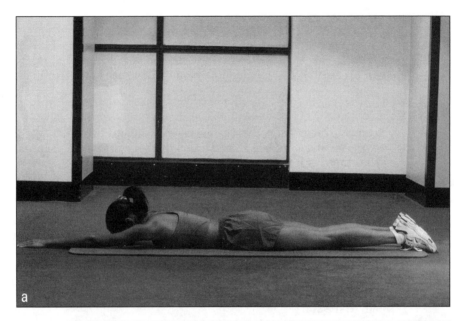

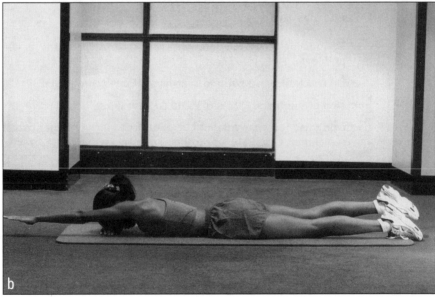

Figure 11-9:
Stretch out as you perform opposite extensions.

Partial roll-up

Purpose: This exercise works your abdominals. Strong abs are essential for upright walking posture and for keeping the lower back in proper alignment.

Lower back, neck

Setup: Lie on your back with your knees bent and "zipped" together. Extend your arms straight out behind you on the floor with your palms facing each other. (See Figure 11-10a.)

Pull your abdominals gently inward.

Movement: Leading with your fingertips, reach your arms to the ceiling, tuck your chin to your chest, pull your abdominals in even more, and peel your spine off the floor by curling upward and forward, as shown in Figure 11-10a. How high you lift depends upon how strong and flexible your spine is: You will probably be able to clear the bottom of your shoulder blades off the floor. Hold a moment at the top of the movement and slowly retrace your path to the start.

Do's and Don'ts:

- ✔ Do imagine that you are moving one vertebra at a time as you both lift and lower.
- ✔ Do reach forward with your arms as you lift and lower.
- ✔ Don't hunch your shoulders up to your ears.
- ✔ Don't use jerky movements in an effort to lift yourself up farther. The movement should be controlled and precise.
- ✔ Don't allow your feet to pop up off the floor. If this happens, you are trying to lift up farther than your abdominal strength will allow.

Modifications:

- ✔ **Full roll-up:** This is a very challenging modification. Roll all the way up to a sitting position and reach your arms forward and slightly upward to sit up tall. Slowly curl down to the start.
- ✔ **Modified roll-up:** To make this exercise easier, straighten your legs a few inches and place your feet hip-width apart. When you hit your "sticking point," place your hands underneath your thighs and gently assist yourself upward.

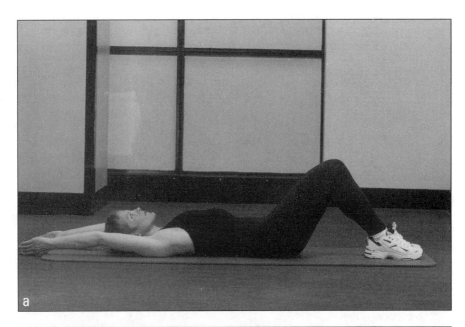

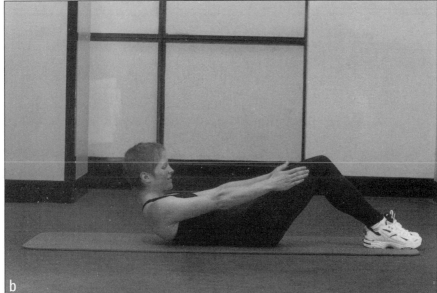

Figure 11-10:
Keep your
abs tight
with the
partial
roll-up.

The golden rules of weight training

Rest for 30 to 90 seconds between exercises. When you're first starting out, you need to rest more between sets. As you get in better shape, you can and should decrease your between-set rest to pump up the intensity of your workout.

Remember to breathe. Exhale through your mouth when you are exerting an effort and inhale through your nose when you are releasing the effort. For example, when you do the partial roll up exercise described in this chapter, exhale as you curl up and inhale as you lower down.

Lift slowly. Never use quick, jerky, or sloppy movements in an attempt to move a weight through an exercise. Here's a good, safe rule: Take two slow counts to lift a weight and four slow counts to lower it.

Use the proper amount of weight. If you can't do at least 8 reps without breaking form, decrease the weight. On the other hand, once you can do more than 15 reps without breaking a sweat or feeling any fatigue in the targeted muscles, you must increase the weight. Pay attention to this rule because it's vital to your progress. You will probably use a different weight for each exercise, and over time, you will need to gradually increase the amount of weight you use.

Use proper form. Read the exercise descriptions carefully and follow them to the letter. *How* you do each exercise is more important than which exercises you do, how many you do, or how much weight you use.

Chapter 12

Stretches for Walkers

· ·

· ·

Almost all aerobics instructors, personal trainers, and fitness experts recommend regular stretching to keep muscles loose and limber, ease muscle soreness, and prevent injury. Yet surprisingly, the American College of Sports Medicine (ACSM), a respected health organization, didn't issue guidelines for stretching exercises until late 1995.

Perhaps the ACSM, along with many other organizations, was slow to offer a road map for flexibility training because no one completely understands what stretching does. Little research exists to support the benefits of stretching, and some studies that have been done are inconclusive.

A few studies even make a compelling case for skipping flexibility work altogether. For instance, one study done at the University of Hawaii and Guilford College in Greensboro, North Carolina, found that runners who don't stretch expend less energy and have fewer injuries than those who do. Another study found that some exercisers actually experience increased muscle soreness after stretching.

Usually, I go with the research because I believe that such studies are the best way to weed out trumped-up hype from the real deal. However, when it comes to stretching exercises for walkers, I make an exception. I think stretching is a good idea. Even though no one really understands flexibility very well, I can tell you from experience and intuition that stretching helps you as a walker. When your muscles are more pliable, your stride is certainly looser and easier. Good flexibility also helps you maintain balance, posture, and agility as you get older. Will stretching help prevent muscle soreness and injuries? The research ranges from maybe to no, but certainly many top experts and athletes believe that stretching does work.

Defining Flexibility

Before you can go about improving your flexibility, you need to know what it is. *Flexibility* refers to the range of motion or distance you can move a joint through. For instance, if you can't touch your toes, it's because the hamstring muscles in the backs of your thighs are only able to stretch to a certain length. If they were longer and more pliable, you'd be able to move your hip joint through a greater range of motion in order to touch your toes.

Stretching is the key to maintaining your flexibility. As you get older, your tendons (the tissues that connect muscle to bone) begin to shorten and tighten, restricting your flexibility. Your movement becomes slower and less fluid. You have more trouble standing up as straight. You walk more stiffly and with a shorter stride. You find it more difficult to step up to a curb or bend down to pick up the trash. Stretching your rear thigh, hips, and calf muscles can help keep you supple and your movements more natural even as you get older.

Good flexibility is one of the keys to helping you maintain good posture. If your neck muscles are short and tight, your head angles forward. If your shoulders and chest are tight, your shoulders round inward. If your lower back, rear thigh, and hip muscles are tight, the curve of your back becomes exaggerated. A regular stretching routine also can reduce pain and discomfort, particularly in your lower back. In fact, the pain often disappears when you begin doing simple stretches for your lower back and rear thigh muscles.

The golden rules of stretching

Here are some basic rules to help you do the stretching routine in this chapter effectively and safely.

✔ Hold each of the basic stretch versions for ten slow counts. As you hold, take at least two deep breaths.

✔ Contrary to popular belief, you should not stretch before a workout. Attempting to prod cold, tight muscles into new positions is practically begging for an injury. It's better to stretch after a workout, when muscles are warm and pliable. Active Isolated (AI) stretching is the exception to this rule; because it is movement oriented, it sends blood into the muscles and increases body temperature. Therefore, you can add AI to your warm-up and/or cool-down.

✔ As you slowly move into each basic stretching position, pay attention to how you feel. Focus on the muscles being stretched and try to feel the stretch spread through the muscle.

✔ A proper stretch should rate anywhere from mild tension to the edge of discomfort on your pain meter. It should never cause severe pain in the muscle you're stretching.

✔ Stretch as often as you like, daily if you can. Always stretch after every workout.

✔ Pay particular attention to those muscles that feel overly tight.

What's more, flexibility exercises can correct muscle imbalances. For instance, suppose that your outer thigh muscles are strong, but your inner thighs are tight and weak. Chances are, you won't even notice this, but it will throw off your movement in subtle ways — you may have trouble standing up from a sitting position or bringing your legs together quickly to avoid stepping in a puddle. Muscle imbalances can eventually lead to injuries such as pulled muscles. They also contribute to clumsiness, which in and of itself can lead to injury. Finally, flexibility can help you become a better walker because it helps keep your walking stride effortless and naturally smooth.

Your flexibility depends largely on two factors. Joint structure — the way your joints are put together and how far they can bend and move — accounts for about 45 percent of flexibility. Because your joint structure is largely hereditary, you really can't do much about it. The other 55 percent of your flexibility depends on the condition of muscle fibers and lubrication of the joints. You can improve those factors by performing the stretching routine in this chapter.

My friend Holly Byrne is an ex-dancer. She can practically wrap her leg around her neck, whereas I, as a runner, hiker, and walker, haven't been able to touch my toes since the '70s. Holly's hips, lower back, and hamstrings are limber. It's a bit of an understatement to say mine are not. Even when she was eight months pregnant and couldn't see her toes, she still got closer to her toes than I can to mine.

Being Flexible about Your Stretching Program

If you thought stretching was as simple as bending over and touching your toes, think again. In the last few years, a quiet flexibility revolution has been going on in gyms across the country. Here's a rundown of some of the more popular flexibility methods that you're likely to encounter.

Hold it

When you sit on the floor, reach for your toes and hold that position for 10 to 30 seconds. This stretch is an example of traditional, or static, stretching. The theory behind this type of stretching is that if you hold a stretch long enough, the muscle "remembers" its newly elongated position, and if you repeat this stretch often enough, the muscle eventually becomes more flexible. Holding a stretch for more than 30 seconds may be too much of a good thing and seems to increase your risk of injury while stretching.

✔ **Pros:** This type of stretching is easy to do and recommended by the ACSM. Most moves stretch more than one muscle group at a time.

✔ **Cons:** Static stretching can be uncomfortable for someone who is inflexible to begin with. Isolating individual muscle groups can be difficult.

Bounce

If you've ever seen films of football warm-up drills from the 1950s, you have a good idea of what ballistic stretching looks like: short, quick bounces to release a muscle. This type of stretch is supposed to override the muscle's reflex mechanisms so that you can reach past your normal point of flexibility before the muscle has time to realize what you're doing and attempt to stop you.

✔ **Pros:** This method most closely mimics many kinds of explosive sports movements. A very few studies have found this to be an effective way to increase flexibility while bypassing muscle soreness.

✔ **Cons:** Ballistic stretching poses great potential for injury. Virtually no respectable organizations condone this type of stretching.

Get some assistance

This exercise is officially known as proprioceptive neuromuscular facilitation. How's that for a mouthful? (Save yourself the trouble and refer to it as PNF.) This type of stretching involves a 6-second tightening of the muscle followed by a 10- to 30-second stretch assisted by another person. Here's one example: You lie on your back with your leg resting on top of your trainer's shoulder. Your trainer carefully moves your leg toward your head until you feel a strong stretch through the back of your thigh. Next, you press down on her shoulder for 10 seconds or so and then relax. Your trainer is then able to stretch your leg a little farther. If you don't have a trainer, you can use a towel, rope, or belt to help yourself stretch a little bit farther.

✔ **Pros:** Several studies have shown PNF to yield superior results for some individuals. In addition, having assistance is always nice, especially if you have limited flexibility.

✔ **Cons:** You risk potential for injury if you push a PNF stretch too far.

I once witnessed an unfortunate event in which a trainer leaned all his weight on his client's back while attempting a PNF stretch and tore all her inner thigh muscles. You could hear the pop from across the room.

Two-second stretches

Active Isolated, or AI, stretching relies on the fact that muscles have equal and opposite reactions. By contracting (tightening) the muscle opposite your stretch, your muscle has no choice but to relax and stretch that much farther. Another principle of AI stretching is keeping the stretch short and sweet. By holding a stretch position for no more than 2 seconds, you don't allow the "stretch reflex" to kick in and prevent the muscle from stretching farther. Many of the AI stretches use a rope, towel, or belt to assist the stretch a little farther than you would be able to do on your own. For more detailed information on stretching aids, see the sidebar "Stretching your options," later in this chapter.

- ✔ **Pros:** You can isolate a few muscles at a time. AI stretching is the least painful way to stretch, even for the flexibility challenged.

- ✔ **Cons:** No real research is available to support theories on AI stretching. Some of the positions are difficult to get into.

The CRAC stretch

For a stretch that's sort of a combination of PNF and AI stretching, try CRAC, short for Contract, Relax, And Contract. This is a fairly new stretching technique — at least it's new to the health club scene. It involves stretching a muscle, tightening it, and then tightening the muscle directly opposite it. You wait for about 20 seconds before moving into the next stretch. To stretch the quadriceps muscles in the front of your thighs in this way, start by bending your knee and pulling your heel toward your buttocks for about 10 seconds. Next, tighten your quadriceps as much as possible for the next 10 seconds or so. Finally, relax your quadriceps as you tighten your hamstring muscles (located in the back of your thighs) for about 10 seconds before taking a break.

- ✔ **Pros:** Limited research seems to indicate effectiveness. This stretch is good for isolating muscles and offers some strengthening benefits as well.

- ✔ **Cons:** You need good coordination and a good connection between your brain and muscles to master this stretch. It's best done with a partner.

Which Stretch Is Best?

The ACSM guidelines recommend doing a traditional 10- to 30-second stretch for each often used muscle group, such as the thighs, lower back, and chest. This is the most common type of stretching taught in aerobics classes, although many stretching and flexibility experts take issue with this advice because it doesn't take into account the benefits and ideas of the other stretching methods. So which method will work best for you?

I suggest that you experiment with a combination of static, AI, and — when you're lucky enough to have a partner or trainer — PNF or CRAC stretching. They are all safe and straightforward as long as you are a stickler for form and don't push beyond your limits. Walkers can benefit from doing any of these stretching techniques.

Flexible activities

Walkers and runners are notorious for being antistretch. Whether the reason is boredom, discomfort, or stretch phobia, they simply do not stretch, even if their muscles feel tight or they suffer from frequent muscle pulls. For those who simply won't try stretching on their own, yoga or Pilates classes or private instruction may be a good solution to poor flexibility. Those two options also offer some strength building and stress reduction.

Great as they are, disciplines like yoga and Pilates demand a high degree of flexibility from the get-go and therefore may be rough for those who are flexibility challenged. In addition, the quality of instruction is so uneven. Because no legal or universal requirements have been established for teaching yoga, anyone can call himself a yoga teacher. For more information on this popular discipline, see *Yoga For Dummies* by Georg Feuerstein and Larry Payne (IDG Books Worldwide).

Be sure to get a glowing word-of-mouth recommendation and test out a few yoga or Pilates classes for yourself. A good instructor understands your flexibility limitations and offers plenty of modifications to work around them. A bad instructor can injure you by forcing you into positions that are best left for pretzels and sailor's knots.

By the way, Pilates is a sort of "active," movement-oriented yoga. It is based on an exercise system invented by Joseph Pilates *(puh LAH teez)* about a century ago to help injured dancers get back on their feet. Though Pilates teachers are required to take intensive course work and go through a lengthy internship, many offshoots of Pilates are now available that go by other names. Some of these Pilates-based systems are better than others.

The Method and the Physical Mind Institute are two good incarnations of the Pilates method. I have been taking Method classes with its creator, Jennifer Kries, for about three years, and although no one would ever mistake me for a world-class gymnast, I have made vast improvements in posture and overall flexibility.

Routine stretching

Now, it's time to stretch out those kinks and loosen up those creaky old joints. To this end, I've developed a stretching program that specifically targets the muscles that walkers use, in the way they use them.

I recommend stretching after every walk. Notice that I say *after,* not before. One of the most enduring myths in exercise is that you should stretch before exercise. In fact, this is the worst time to stretch because that's when your muscles are at their coldest and tightest. At the very least, you should warm up by walking at a moderately brisk pace for at least 5 minutes before you stretch to get your blood pumping and to elevate your body temperature. (Active Isolated stretching is the only exception here; because it's movement oriented, you can use it as a warm-up.)

For your convenience, I organize these stretches so that they go from standing to lying on the floor rather than from head to toe. This order makes it easier for you to zip through the routine. You should feel comfortable with the stretching positions and your particular flexibility quirks after only a few stretching sessions. After you're familiar with the routine, you can probably complete it in about 10 minutes. (For more detailed stretching technique tips, see the sidebar "The Golden Rules of Stretching," earlier in this chapter.)

I include an AI alternative stretch for every static stretch in the routine in this chapter because I find it a more comfortable way to stretch. I am not flexible by nature, so I find that even basic stretching positions are just too uncomfortable to hold for that slow count of 10. However, I can bear the 2-second mini-stretches that are an integral part of AI.

At some point, try both the traditional and AI versions of each stretch. You may find that you like the static version of one stretch and the AI version of another.

Neck stretch

This stretch (shown in Figure 12-1) eases tension in your neck and upper shoulders.

Stretch: With your shoulders down and relaxed, drop your left ear toward your left shoulder. Hold for 10 slow counts and then repeat to the right. You may place your left hand on your right ear to gently assist the stretch.

You'll feel the stretch at the base of your neck, and the stretch will gradually travel upward.

Do's:

- ✔ Do keep your shoulders down and relaxed.
- ✔ Do stretch your right arm down and away to increase the stretch.

AI alternative: Do the same move by using your left hand to gently assist the stretch. Hold for 2 slow counts, repeat 8 to 15 times, and then repeat to the left side.

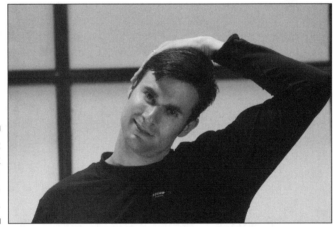

Figure 12-1:
The neck stretch helps ease tension.

Chest expansion

This stretch (see Figure 12-2) targets your shoulders, chest, and arms, the muscles that power your arm swing as you walk and that also have a key role in proper posture.

Stretch: In a tall sitting or standing position, reach your arms behind you and clasp your hands together. Lift your chest up even higher, raise your arms up slightly, and hold for 10 slow counts. Repeat 2 to 3 times.

As you hold the position, you will feel a mild stretch spread across your chest, through the front of your shoulders, and down the front of your arms.

Shoulders, elbows

Don'ts:

- ✔ Don't force your arms up higher than is comfortable.
- ✔ Don't hunch your shoulders up to your ears.
- ✔ Don't arch your lower back.

AI alternative: This alternative is good if you have limited shoulder flexibility. Stand tall and reach your straight arms back behind you, keeping your elbows locked and your palms facing towards each other. Hold for 2 slow counts and then swing your arms forward before beginning the next repetition. Repeat 8 to 15 times.

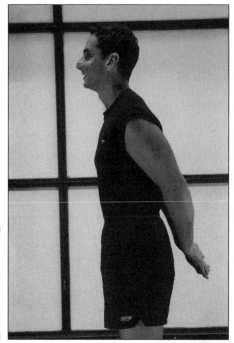

Figure 12-2:
You can do the chest expansion sitting or standing.

Hamstring stretch

The hamstring stretch is a great stretch for your hamstrings and your lower back, two muscles that tend to feel tight after walking.

Stretch: Stand tall with your left foot a few inches in front of your right foot and your left toe lifted. Pull your abdominals gently inward, lean forward from your hips, and rest both palms on top of your right thigh for balance and support. Keep your shoulders down and relaxed; don't round your lower back. Hold this position for 10 slow counts. Repeat the stretch with your right leg forward. (Figure 12-3 shows this version of the hamstring stretch.)

You should feel a mild pull gradually spread throughout the back of your leg as you hold this stretch.

Lower back

Don'ts:

- ✔ Don't lean so far forward that you lose your balance.
- ✔ Don't push the stretch to the point that you feel strain in your lower back.

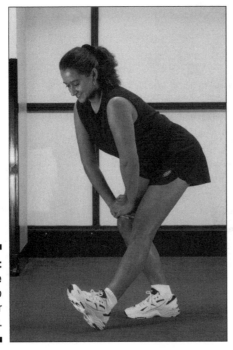

Figure 12-3:
Here's one way to stretch your hamstrings.

AI alternative: Try this stretch (shown in Figure 12-4) if you have chronic lower back problems or you find it uncomfortable to hold your hamstrings in the stretched position. Lie on your back with your left knee bent, foot flat on the floor. Loop your rope, towel, or belt around the instep of your right foot and hold an end in each hand. Straighten your right leg up as high and as far as you comfortably can. Tighten the front of your thigh and hold for 2 slow counts before bending your right knee to release the stretch. Repeat 8 to 15 times and then stretch with your left leg.

Figure 12-4:
Use this alternative hamstring stretch if you have lower back problems.

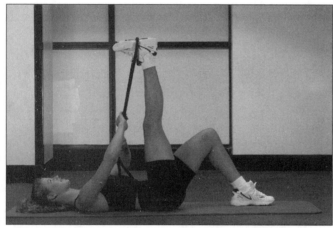

Quad stretch

This stretch (see Figure 12-5) focuses on the *quadriceps* (front of thigh) muscles, which can feel tight and tired after a walking workout.

Stretch: Stand tall with your feet hip-width apart. Hold on to a chair or the wall if you need support. Bend your left leg so that your heel moves toward your buttocks and grasp your foot in your right hand. Hold for 10 slow counts and then stretch your right leg.

You should feel a mild pull gradually spread throughout the front of your leg as you hold this stretch.

Knee, lower back

Do's and don'ts:

✔ Do remember to keep your abdominals pulled in and your shoulders back.

✔ Don't lock the knee of your base leg.

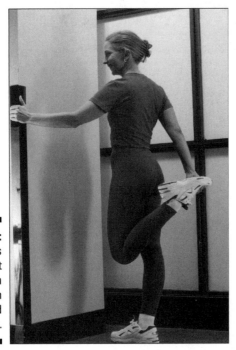

Figure 12-5:
The muscles in the front of your thigh benefit from the quad stretch.

AI alternative: Try this if you are prone to knee problems or find it hard to do the basic version of this stretch. Lie on your left side with your knees curled into your chest. Rest your head on your left arm and grasp your left shin with your left hand. Keeping your right knee bent, tighten your hamstring and buttocks and gently pull your leg back as far as you can. Hold for 2 slow counts and release. Repeat 8 to 15 times and then stretch with your left leg.

Calf stretch

Good walking form involves lifting the toe and planting the foot, movements that can tire out the muscles in your lower legs. The calf stretch (shown in Figure 12-6) offers some relief for the calves.

Stretch: Stand tall and face a wall about 2 feet away. Straddle your legs so that your right leg is forward and slightly bent and your left leg is behind and as straight as possible. Pull your abdominals gently inward and don't round your lower back. With straight arms, press your palms into the wall and lean forward. Hold for 10 slow counts and then repeat the stretch on the other side to stretch your right calf.

You should feel a mild stretch spread throughout your calf as you hold the stretch.

Do's:

- ✔ Do keep both heels flat on the floor.
- ✔ Do keep your back leg completely straight so that you get the best stretch.

Figure 12-6:
Help ease tired lower leg muscles with the calf stretch.

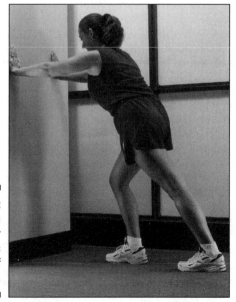

AI alternative: This stretches both the shins and the calves. Sit on the floor with both legs straight out in front of you. Holding an end of the rope in each hand, loop the rope around the instep of your right foot, and bend your left knee slightly. Flex your right foot back, pointing your toes towards your knee and using the rope to gently assist you a little further. Hold for 2 slow counts, point your toe, repeat the stretch 8 to 15 times, and then stretch your left calf.

Cat-Cow

This movement stretches your abdominals and lower back, two areas that may tire out after a walk. Figure 12-7 demonstrates how to do this stretch.

Stretch: Kneel on your hands and knees so that your knees are directly under your hips and your hands are directly under your shoulders. Pull your abdominals inward and gently round your back upward. Hold for 5 slow counts and then gently arch your back downward and hold for 5 slow counts. Repeat 1 to 3 times.

When you round your back, you should feel a mild stretch through your lower back. When you arch your back, you should feel a stretch in both your abdominals and lower back.

Lower back

Do's and don'ts:

- ✔ Do limit the range of movement if you feel lower back discomfort.
- ✔ Don't hunch your shoulders up toward your ears.
- ✔ Don't lean so far forward that you lose your balance.

AI alternative: This stretches your abdominals and lower back. Sit up tall on the floor with your knees bent, hold your hands just underneath your knees, and point your toes slightly upward. Tuck your chin toward your chest, gently pull your abdominals inward, and round your upper body forward toward your feet. (Use your arms to assist you.) Hold for 2 slow counts and then slowly restraighten your back. Repeat 8 to 15 times.

Figure 12-7:
The cat-cow works on your abdominals and lower back.

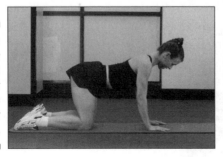 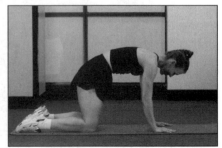

Sun salutation

This move (see Figure 12-8) stretches your entire upper body as well as your torso and front hip and thigh muscles.

Stretch: Kneel on the floor and bring your left leg forward so that your knee is bent, your left foot is flat on the floor, and your left thigh is parallel to the floor. Place your hands on top of your left thigh for balance. Pull your abdominals gently inward and keep your shoulders down and back. Stretch upward as you lean slightly forward. Hold for 10 seconds. Repeat with the right leg forward.

You'll feel this stretch travel through your torso and upper body, including your arms. You'll also feel it at the very top of the back thigh.

Lower back

Do's and don'ts:

- ✔ Do hold on to something solid with one hand if you have trouble maintaining balance.
- ✔ Don't lean so far forward that your front knee moves in front of your toes.
- ✔ Don't arch your lower back.

AI alternative: Try this stretch if you have trouble getting into or out of the basic sun salutation stretch or if your front hip and thigh muscles are exceptionally tight. Stand tall with your feet hip-width apart. Raise your right arm upward directly in line with your shoulder and extend your left arm down. Stretch both arms in opposite directions as if you are trying to touch the ceiling and the floor, respectively. Hold for 2 counts and then switch arm positions. Continue alternating until you have completed 8 to 15 reps with each arm up.

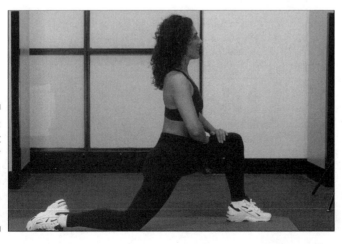

Figure 12-8:
Be sure not to arch your back when doing the sun salutation.

Butterfly

This exercise (shown in Figure 12-9) stretches your inner thighs, hips, and lower back muscles.

Stretch: Sit up tall with the soles of your feet pressed together and your knees dropped to the sides as far as they will comfortably go. Pull your abdominals gently inward and lean forward from your hips. Grasp your feet with your hands and carefully pull yourself slightly farther forward. Hold for 10 slow counts. Repeat 2 to 3 times.

As you hold this position, you'll feel the stretch spread throughout your inner thighs, the outermost part of your hips, and your lower back.

Lower back

Do's and don'ts:

- ✔ Do increase the stretch by carefully pressing your thighs toward the floor as you hold the position.
- ✔ Don't hunch your shoulders up toward your ears.
- ✔ Don't round your lower back.

AI alternative: Try this stretch if you lack overall hip and thigh flexibility or find it uncomfortable to hold an inner thigh stretch position. Lie on your back with your legs together and your rope looped around the instep of your right foot. Thread the rope under the inside of your right ankle so that both ends of the rope are on the outside of your right calf; grasp both ends in your right hand and completely straighten both of your legs. Using the rope to gently assist you and leading with your heel, move your right leg a few inches away from the midline of your body until you feel a mild stretch through your inner thigh. Hold for 2 slow counts, repeat 8 to 15 times, and then repeat the stretch with your left leg.

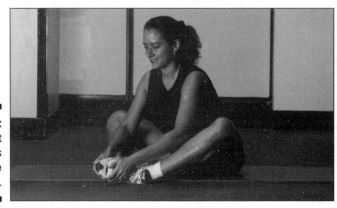

Figure 12-9:
You don't
need wings
to do the
butterfly.

Pretzel

Many walkers feel tightness in their outer hips. This stretch (demonstrated in Figure 12-10) pinpoints that area.

Stretch: Lie on your back with your left knee bent, your left foot flat on the floor, and your right ankle resting across the top of your left thigh. With your legs in this position, lift them up so that your left thigh is perpendicular to the floor. Clasp your hands around your left thigh and gently pull it back toward you. Hold for 10 slow counts. Repeat the stretch with your right knee bent.

You'll feel a stretch spread throughout your buttocks and hips as you hold this position.

Do's and Don'ts:

- ✔ Don't hunch your shoulders up toward your ears.
- ✔ Do lift your head up off the floor if it feels more comfortable.

AI alternative: Try this stretch if you have extremely tight hips and have trouble getting into the pretzel position. Sit tall in a chair with your left foot flat on the floor and your right ankle resting on your left thigh. Place your right hand on your right knee and your left hand on your right ankle. Keeping your back straight and your abdominals gently pulled inward, lean forward from the hips and gently press your right knee toward the floor with your hand. Hold for 2 slow counts and release. Repeat 8 to 15 times and then stretch your left side.

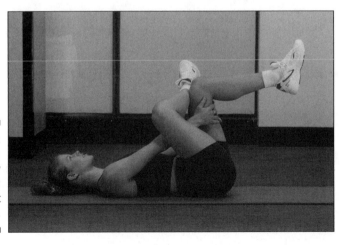

Figure 12-10:
You can see how the pretzel stretch got its name.

Knee hug

Your lower back and buttocks can get tight and tired after a walk, especially if you've been focusing on your posture. This stretch (see Figure 12-11) serves as a mild, yet effective, back and hip release.

Stretch: Lie on your back with your knees bent in toward your chest. Hold your hands underneath your thighs and pull your thighs even closer to your chest. Hold for 10 slow counts. Repeat 2 to 3 times.

You will feel a mild stretch through your buttocks and lower back.

Do's and don'ts:

✔ Do bring your head up toward your knees if that feels more comfortable.

✔ Don't hunch your shoulders up toward your ears.

✔ Don't allow your lower back to lift up off the floor.

AI alternative: Try this stretch if you have an exceptionally tight lower back or find it uncomfortable to hold the stretch. Do this stretch exactly the same way you do the basic stretch, but hold it for only 2 slow counts before releasing. Repeat 8 to 15 times.

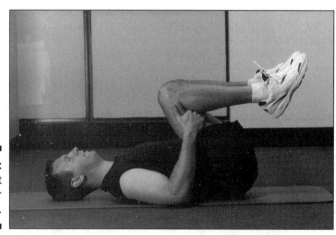

Figure 12-11:
Don't forget
to hug your
knees.

Stretching your options

Many Active Isolated stretches call for the aid of a special rope to help assist and guide you through the movement. If your flexibility is limited, you may also want to consider using the rope or another stretching aid. For instance, some people don't have enough shoulder and chest flexibility to clasp their hands behind their back as called for in the chest expansion stretch in this chapter. Reaching behind and holding the end of a rope in each hand is a very effective modification. I recommend purchasing one of the following products if you plan on doing the Active Isolated (AI) stretches or you want that extra bit of help. (Ordering information is included in the appendix.)

✔ **AI Stretch Rope:** This long, thick, black rope is designed especially for AI stretching and costs about $10. I've also seen it used in yoga classes. You can find it in some yoga catalogs and in the wonderful *Health for Life* catalog.

✔ **Stretch Rite:** To use this nylon belt with giant beads, you reach as far as you can and hold on between two beads. As you hold the stretch, you can gradually creep your hands forward to the next set of beads. This product is available in the *Health for Life* catalog and costs about $20. You can find the information on this catalog in the appendix.

✔ **The Stretch Out Strap:** This long rubber strap has a series of loops along its spine. The loops are great for looping your hands and feet through. It's available through the *Health for Life* catalog for about $20.

✔ **Towel or belt:** These items are low-tech, low-cost alternatives to the above gadgets. Make sure that your towel or belt is long enough. If you are sitting or lying on the floor and you loop the center around your instep and straighten your leg, you should be able to hold an end in each hand without compromising your form.

Chapter 13

Advanced Walking Routines

. . . .

In This Chapter

▶ Discovering interval training for speed

▶ Trying some sample speed routines

▶ Upping your tempo

▶ Incorporating more fun into your workouts

. . . .

*W*alking for the sake of walking is a good fitness activity for most people, especially if the goal of the program is to get in shape and lose weight. But at some time, that goal may not be enough for you, even if you experiment with the upper levels of walking. For example, walkers who want to enter a few road races may want a way to increase their competitive edge. And those looking for other ways to spice things up may want to add to their bag of training tricks.

The methods and systems that I describe in this chapter are considered advanced because they give you ways to vary your walking program in other ways besides shifting between the various walking levels. In fact, many of the techniques in this chapter may help you move up to the next level if you have been having trouble doing so. They also add a bit of fun and interest to your walking workouts.

Top athletes of all types have used many of the techniques in this chapter for decades. Some of them have been used for centuries. Must you include them in your walking program? Certainly not. But will you find them useful, challenging, and interesting if you do decide to introduce some or all of them into your workouts? Absolutely. So if you have a competitive spirit — or just a curious soul — give 'em a try.

Interval Training for Speed

Interval training refers to walks that include periods of high-intensity training interspersed with periods of lower-intensity training, or active rest. Active rest is more effective than just stopping and catching your breath after an all-out effort. When you keep moving, your muscles recover faster because your blood keeps flowing through them, speeding nutrients in and taking away the body's waste products produced by high-intensity training.

Interval training has a place in your training if you're looking to compete, spice up your workouts to prevent boredom, burn more calories in a shorter period of time, or kick up your speed a notch. Interval training works best when done at Level 3, high-energy walking (see Chapter 9), or Level 4, walk-run (see Chapter 10). In fact, walk-run is a form of interval training in and of itself.

In interval training, you can vary the following three factors, which change depending on your goals and abilities:

- ✔ The total time and/or distance of each hard and easy interval
- ✔ The number of intervals you perform
- ✔ The frequency of your interval training workouts

Time and distance of hard and easy intervals

The total time of each hard interval and each active rest interval depends on what you're trying to achieve. (The distance you travel varies depending on how fast you walk.)

- ✔ **Wind sprints lasting from 10 to 45 seconds help improve your sprinting speed.** They're the adult equivalent of the 50-yard dash you used to do in high school gym class. They're quick, intense, and leave you gasping for breath at the end.

  This is a great type of training to include in your workouts if you are planning to compete or you like the feeling of very high-intensity training. You alternate sprints with active rest periods of 10 to 45 seconds. Attempt this type of training only if you're an experienced walker with a good-to-excellent fitness level.

- ✔ **"Lactic acid training" intervals lasting from 60 to 90 seconds alternated with equal to double the amount of rest train the body's lactic acid systems.** Training this way helps you build up tolerance to lactic acid so that you can train harder and faster. It's a good way to work out when you're trying to move up to the next level in terms of overall walking speed.

Without getting into too much science and jargon, *lactic acid* is a substance that is created during your body's chemical reactions used to produce energy for movement. When you exercise very hard for short periods of time, lactic acid floods into your muscles, inhibiting energy production and causing a burning, painful sensation in your muscles. As a result, you either have to stop or slow down in order to allow your body to flush this excess lactic acid from the muscles.

✔ **Aerobic intervals of 2 to 5 minutes improve your ability to process oxygen and therefore help increase endurance.** Recovery intervals are usually equal to or greater than hard intervals. This is a great type of training for a greater calorie burn and to help you pick up your typical walking pace.

The shorter the speed interval, the faster your speed. For example, you will not be able to walk at the same speed for 2 minutes as you will for 10 seconds, so don't even try. The object is to pick a speed that is challenging for the length of the interval you're performing. Regardless of the length and absolute speed of each interval, all intervals should feel challenging under the circumstances.

A good way to measure the intensity of each interval is to use your heart rate, the rating of perceived exertion scale, or the talk test. I describe all these methods in Chapter 5.

In general, the newer you are to high-intensity interval training, the longer your active rest periods need to be. When you first begin interval training, start with the greatest amount of recommended rest possible. In fact, rest as long as you need. Gradually over time, you will need shorter and shorter rest periods to recover and move into the next interval.

The number of intervals you perform

Interval training is high intensity by definition. As a result, you will be sore after your first two or three interval training walks. Ideally, you can minimize this soreness to a pleasant ache that goes away after a few days. I have clients who jump into interval training with a bit too much gusto. As a result, they can't even shuffle their feet the next day, let alone go for another walk.

I recommend starting out with five to six high-intensity intervals during a 30- to 60-minute time period. Increase by one additional interval a week per interval workout until you can do eight to ten intervals without feeling exhausted or sore after your workout. After you get to this higher level, you can start adding in other types of intervals or a greater number of aerobic intervals. You can mix and match the type of intervals you do within a workout, depending on your goals and preferences. Always do a 5- to 10-minute warm-up and a 5- to 10-minute cool-down to start and finish your interval workout.

Frequency of interval training workouts

Start out with one interval training walk a week. You may find that one such session is plenty.

Don't do more than three interval training sessions a week. Overdoing any type of high-intensity training carries the risk of injury and burnout.

You can perform your interval training anywhere, but it is most effective when performed on a track or a treadmill. Both of these venues make it easy to keep track of time and distance. Plus they are both flat and even.

Sample Speed Interval Routines

I provide some sample interval routines to try in Tables 13-1 through 13-5. Try the beginner interval training routine first and then explore your comfort level by trying some of the others. You need not progress beyond aerobic interval training unless you have specific competitive or speed goals. However, you may find lactic acid and wind sprint intervals fun to do and a good way to get a fast and furious workout when you don't have tons of time.

Table 13-1	Beginner Interval Training Routine	
Interval	*Intensity*	*Time*
Warm-up	Easy	5 minutes
Interval 1	Challenging	2 minutes
Active rest 1	Easy	3 minutes
Interval 2	Challenging	2 minutes
Active rest 2	Easy	3 minutes
Interval 3	Challenging	2 minutes
Active rest 3	Easy	3 minutes
Interval 4	Challenging	2 minutes
Active rest 4	Easy	3 minutes
Interval 5	Challenging	2 minutes
Cool-down	Easy	5 minutes
Total walk time		32 minutes

Table 13-2	Advanced Aerobic Interval Training Routine	
Interval	*Intensity*	*Time*
Warm-up	Easy	5 minutes
Interval 1	Challenging	2 minutes
Active rest 1	Easy	3 minutes
Interval 2	Challenging	3 minutes
Active rest 2	Easy	3 minutes
Interval 3	Challenging	4 minutes
Active rest 3	Easy	3 minutes
Interval 4	Challenging	5 minutes
Active rest 4	Easy	3 minutes
Interval 5	Challenging	4 minutes
Active rest 5	Easy	3 minutes
Interval 6	Challenging	3 minutes
Active rest 6	Easy	3 minutes
Interval 7	Challenging	2 minutes
Active rest 7	Easy	3 minutes
Interval 8	Challenging	5 minutes
Cool-down	Easy	5 minutes
Total walk time		59 minutes

Table 13-3	Basic Wind Sprint Interval Training Routine	
Interval	*Intensity*	*Time*
Warm-up	Easy	5 minutes
Interval 1	Challenging	45 seconds
Active rest 1	Easy	45 seconds
Interval 2	Challenging	30 seconds
Active rest 2	Easy	30 seconds
Interval 3	Challenging	10 seconds
Active rest 3	Easy	10 seconds
Interval 4	Challenging	30 seconds
Active rest 4	Easy	30 seconds
Interval 5	Challenging	45 seconds
Cool-down	Easy	5 minutes
Total walk time		Approximately 15 minutes

Note: As your fitness level improves and you want more of a challenge, repeat the entire interval sequence two to three times before cooling down.

Table 13-4	Basic Lactic Acid Interval Training Routine	
Interval	*Intensity*	*Time*
Warm-up	Easy	5 minutes
Interval 1	Challenging	1 minute
Active rest 1	Easy	2 minutes
Interval 2	Challenging	1 minute
Active rest 2	Easy	2 minutes
Interval 3	Challenging	1 minute
Active rest 3	Easy	2 minutes
Interval 4	Challenging	2 minutes
Active rest 4	Easy	2 minutes
Interval 5	Challenging	2 minutes
Cool-down	Easy	5 minutes
Total walk time		25 minutes

Note: As your fitness level improves, you can make this workout more challenging by repeating the entire interval sequence two to three times before cooling down.

Table 13-5	Mix and Match Interval Training Routine	
Interval	*Intensity*	*Time*
Warm-up	Easy	5 minutes
Interval 1	Challenging	30 seconds
Active rest 1	Easy	30 seconds
Interval 2	Challenging	1 minute
Active rest 2	Easy	1 minute
Interval 3	Challenging	2 minutes
Active rest 3	Easy	2 minutes
Interval 4	Challenging	3 minutes
Active rest 4	Easy	3 minutes
Interval 5	Challenging	4 minutes
Active rest 5	Easy	4 minutes
Interval 6	Challenging	5 minutes
Active rest 6	Easy	5 minutes
Interval 7	Challenging	4 minutes
Active rest 7	Easy	4 minutes
Interval 8	Challenging	3 minutes
Active rest 8	Easy	3 minutes
Interval 9	Challenging	2 minutes
Active rest 9	Easy	2 minutes
Interval 10	Challenging	1 minute
Active rest 10	Easy	1 minute
Interval 11	Challenging	30 seconds
Cool-down	Easy	5 minutes
Total time		Approximately 57 minutes

Tempo Training

Allegro is an Italian word that any music buff recognizes as instruction to quicken the speed at which you play a musical piece. It's also an apt way to describe *tempo training*. Instead of doing brief bursts at all-out speeds, as with traditional interval training, tempos involve moving at moderately challenging paces for long stretches. In effect, you hit the high notes and hold 'em like Kenny G.

Tempo training intervals usually last from 8 to 20 minutes. If you are thinking about racing, then do these intervals at race pace speed. Even if you're not thinking about racing, tempo training can still benefit you by building stamina, strength, and speed. Because you go farther and faster, you also burn a greater number of calories in a shorter period of time. All levels of walkers can experiment with tempo training. Doing some tempo training at one level of walking is a good way to make the transition into the next higher level of walking.

Do tempos at about 80 percent of your all-out effort. You're moving at the correct speed when you feel like you're exercising right at the outer edges of your comfort zone: Your breathing is quick and heavy but not ragged; your heart is pounding but not hammering; your muscles are pumping, but you don't "feel the burn."

You can add tempos into your routine once or twice a week. But be careful how you combine them with more traditional interval training. For example, if you are already doing two interval workouts a week, one tempo walk a week will suffice. If you choose to forgo the shorter, speedier intervals, then you can tempo train up to three times a week.

As always, start out conservatively. Never skip your warm-up or cool-down. Start with one 8-minute tempo walk, take an equal amount of rest, and then, if you're up for it, tack on one more 8-minute tempo interval. Over time, you can gradually increase either the number of tempos you perform or the length of each tempo interval.

Adding Play to Your Workouts

For years, I've watched a group of about ten walkers make a game out of their workouts. For instance, sometimes they walk single file, and after a minute or two, the person in the back of the line has to hightail it up to the leadership position. Every few minutes someone calls out, and they switch leaders until everyone has had a turn at the front. I've never spoken to them, but I don't think they're part of any formal group. They just seem to be having fun with their workouts and with each other.

You can use dozens of tricks to make your training more challenging and more interesting without getting into a more formal interval training program. Some, like the follow-the-leader exercise I describe in the preceding anecdote, can only be done when you walk in a group. Most training exercises work fine whether you walk alone or with others.

Fartlek

This charming word means *speed play* in Swedish. It refers to a system in which you walk fast when you feel like it and slower when you feel like it. A Swedish Olympic track coach devised it in 1948.

Fartlek training is not a way to avoid training hard. It's a way to avoid monotony and repetition. Fartleks offer a way to introduce some joy and spontaneity into your tougher walking workouts.

I once did a long walk-run with my husband and a friend near our vacation house in upstate New York. Every so often, we all sped up and tried to keep up with each other for several minutes. Then one of us slowed down. When we came to a stream, we splashed through it. We soared down hills and surged up them. We jogged slowly when we came to some particularly pretty scenery that we wanted to enjoy. We laughed and joked a lot. Although it was a hard, sweaty workout, it seemed to pass in the blink of an eye. This is a classic example of fartlek training at its best.

To add some fartlek into your training, simply walk faster for untimed intervals whenever you feel like it. Throw in faster intervals whenever and how often you like. Don't worry about formally tracking anything. Fartlek works for all levels of walking and is especially useful when you're transitioning up a level.

Telephone pole training

After warming up for 5 minutes or so, walk the distance between two telephone poles at a challenging pace. Then walk at an easy pace between two telephone poles. Keep alternating like this for the entire workout until you're ready for your cool-down.

Telephone pole training is a fun way to do something different even if you don't change your walking route or distance. You don't have to use telephone poles either. I sometimes use bushes or a type of tree, even if they aren't spaced a regular distance apart. In New York City, most city blocks are a tenth of a mile, so I alternate fast and slow blocks. You'll be surprised how quickly this technique makes time go by.

Catch up

Pick a person in the distance and try to catch up to that person. Or try not to let anyone pass you during your walk. If someone does, keep up with that person as long as you can.

I have to admit that I hate when someone else uses me as her rabbit. Because I have a competitive nature, I feel a need to pass the person who has just passed me. Whenever I hear footsteps behind me that seem to be catching up, I put on the gas. This has led to some interesting speed duels with total strangers. Often they last for miles.

This method of speed training works well if, like me, you're a competitor at heart. It gives you something to think about and a visible goal to shoot for during your workout. After you pass someone, start looking for your next victim to mow down.

Counting steps

Counting steps is a great workout when you're out on the road and want to do some structured interval training but don't have a stopwatch or an idea of measured distances. Start out by walking 10 paces hard, followed by 10 paces easy. (A pace equals one full left and right stride.) Next, increase to 20 hard and 20 easy. Increase the length of your intervals until you reach 100 steps hard/easy. When you reach 100 paces, you can take a break for a minute or two to catch your breath. Or, if you want to really push yourself, decrease the number of paces 10 paces at a time until you work yourself down to 10 hard/easy paces once again.

Backward walking

You've probably seen joggers or walkers in your local park turned around and moving backward. Usually they're looking over their shoulder trying not to fall flat on their backs. Are they simply an accident waiting to happen, or does walking backward offer any benefit?

There is no simple answer. Physical therapists often have their patients do some backward walking because it places less pressure on the kneecaps than walking forward. Some studies suggest that turning things around can bump your calorie burn up by as much as 119 percent.

But is it a practical way to work out on a regular basis? Probably not. You don't have eyes in back of your head; therefore, you probably weren't designed to walk backward efficiently or comfortably. Most people can't walk as fast or as far when *retro walking,* as those in the know call it.

Adding a few minutes of backward walking at the end of each workout doesn't do you any harm and may do you some good if you tend to have achy knees. If you retro walk on a treadmill, use the slowest speed possible and hold on lightly to the side rail. If you retro walk outdoors, don't do it in an area fraught with potholes and pitfalls. And definitely don't do what I once tried on a dare: retro walk with your eyes closed. I have the scars to prove what a bad idea that is!

Chapter 14

Advice for Special Needs

*T*hough walking is a form of exercise that virtually everyone can do, the basic rules don't apply to everyone. Some groups of people, like the ones I describe in this chapter, have special considerations to take into account to ensure that they can walk safely and effectively.

If you fall into one of these categories or know someone who does, I urge you to read the sections of this chapter that apply. I let you know how you can walk through your pregnancy and how you can walk for fitness and fun as you age. Finally, if you are one of the millions of people who walk with their dog as your — and his — primary form of exercise, I tell you how to make exercise a safe and enjoyable proposition for both of you.

Walking through Pregnancy

Until the 1980s, there was a common belief that pregnancy should be a period of confinement. Nowadays, the only one who is confined is the baby in its mother's belly. Pregnant women exercising is a common sight, and one of the most common forms of exercise these women engage in is walking.

The benefits of a walking program are still relevant during pregnancy. And doctors now place fewer restrictions on pregnant women who exercise than ever before. For instance, until recently, the American College of Obstetricians and Gynecologists (ACOG) insisted that a pregnant woman should not let her heart rate exceed 140 beats per minute and that she should not exercise for more than 15 minutes at a time. Many fit women found these rules too restrictive. The new ACOG guidelines, released in 1995, eliminated the heart rate and time restrictions and made many pregnant walkers happy.

But the change in ACOG's policy doesn't mean that every pregnant woman can or should exercise without restriction. Every pregnancy is unique, so you need to work with your physician to set up personal guidelines. Most doctors encourage women to continue walking through pregnancy unless there is a legitimate reason not to.

Tips for pregnant walkers

If you were walking before your pregnancy, you can probably continue walking right up to the day you give birth. I have several friends who were in the middle of brisk walks when their water broke. The following tips are some general guidelines for walking and exercising while pregnant. Use them to modify your walking and exercise program, but always check with your doctor for personalized recommendations.

- ✔ **Because your heart rate is affected by so many factors, it's not always the best indicator of how hard you're working during pregnancy, so focus on your** *perceived exertion,* **a fancy word for "how you feel."** (See Chapter 5 for more details on this term.) Rate yourself on a scale of 1 to 10 and try to maintain a workout level that keeps you between 4 and 8. You'll probably find that it takes a lot less exercise to bring you up to that level than before you were pregnant, but because you're exercising for two, that's to be expected! There are no specific guidelines on the length of your workout. Timing should be based on your pre-pregnancy workouts and your doctor's recommendations.

- ✔ **Don't measure your performance against your pre-pregnancy fitness.** You are exercising for two, hauling around a lot of extra weight, and have an off-kilter center of gravity. Don't push yourself to the point of exhaustion. Give yourself permission to take breaks and cut your walk a little short if you're feeling tired.

- ✔ **If you walk on a treadmill, be extremely cautious.** Because your center of gravity is much lower while you're pregnant, your sense of balance may not be up to snuff. You may want to hold onto the handrail lightly when you walk, especially during the latter stages of pregnancy.

- ✔ **After the first trimester (that's after 3 months), don't do any exercises that call for you to lie on your back.** You don't want to compromise blood flow to the baby or run the risk of elevating your blood pressure. You have to forgo exercises like crunches, but you can still do abdominal strengthening exercises from a standing position, leaning against a large ball, or with your back pressed against a wall.

- ✔ **Never push a stretch beyond the point of mild discomfort and don't hold stretches longer than 20 seconds.** Because you have to produce more of the hormone relaxin when you're pregnant, your joints are a little bit looser than usual, and pushing your stretches too far can lead to permanent injuries. Be especially careful when you stretch the muscles that surround your knees, hips, and lower back. However, you should stretch to help relieve general aches and pains.

✔ **Consider purchasing new, well-padded walking shoes for a better fit and to help support your joints.** Your feet may spread and increase by a half to full shoe size as a result of the extra weight they're supporting.

✔ **Weight training is a good form of exercise to continue during pregnancy although pregnancy isn't the best time to start weight training.** Pay special attention to exercises that work your back and shoulders. Keeping these muscles strong helps avoid back and shoulder pains that many women experience during pregnancy, and working these muscles gives you the strength to carry your bundle of joy around after she's born.

✔ **Drink a lot of water before, during, and after your workouts to help keep your system — and the baby's — cool.**

Walking after the baby is born

I can't tell you how many of my clients and readers are surprised when their bodies don't instantly snap back into perfect form as soon as their baby is born. Giving birth is a big event for your body — and that's an understatement. You need to give yourself time to recover and regroup. This is *not* the time to be hard on yourself or negative about your body! I always tell my clients who just gave birth to give themselves at least a year to get back in shape. I strongly suggest skipping any body fat or weight measurements for a while too.

Depending on the complications you may experience during pregnancy, most women can begin fitness walking again within 4 to 6 weeks after giving birth. If you had your baby by caesarean section, you may have to wait a bit longer than that.

Don't expect to start up again at your previous level. But if you walked all through your pregnancy, you can get up to speed very quickly. Use your walking to bond with your baby by taking him out for a spin in the stroller. Baby Jogger makes several models of specially designed strollers for active moms and dads. You can find these strollers in many sporting goods stores or order them through the Road Runner Sports catalog. (See the appendix for contact information.)

Walking When You're Older

What age do you consider old? According to *Modern Maturity Magazine,* people under 30 define old age as beginning at age 63. People ages 30 to 39 define old age as over 67. People ages 40 to 49 define old age as 70 and up. People ages 50 to 59 define old age as over 71. People over 60 define old age as 75 and beyond.

Whatever age you think that it happens upon you, we tend to also have a peculiar way of looking at old age. We think that it's a reason to slow down and take life easy. Many people stop exercising because they think that they're too old and fragile.

Nothing could be further from the truth. Exercise becomes even more important as you age. It preserves bone density and muscle mass. It helps conserve stamina and strength. It improves flexibility and mobility. It boosts mood and keeps you from feeling your age.

At age 75, my mother-in-law is one of the most physically active people I know and one of the most positive, upbeat people I've ever met. "I'm 75 years young!" she often exclaims in her charming Czechoslovakian accent. And it's true. She is one of the "youngest" people you will ever come across. She often credits her daily 1- to 2-hour walks for her ageless energy and stamina.

Getting in the game

There are, however, a few concessions you may need to make to age. For instance, each year after reaching maturity, your heart's ability to pump blood decreases by about 1 percent a year. Your ability to process oxygen also declines by about the same percentage. The number of muscle fibers decreases at a rate of about 3 to 5 percent a year after age 30, leading to a 10- to 30-percent loss of strength by age 60, a lower metabolic rate, and higher body fat. The average 70-year-old has also lost 15 to 30 percent of bone density, a circumstance that results in brittle, easily broken bones.

But recent studies suggest that these declines may be as much a result of inactivity as time. Several large research studies imply that disuse is responsible for as much as 50 percent of functional decline. Most experts believe that these age-associated declines can be delayed, slowed, and even reversed with regular exercise. I am firmly convinced that by engaging in a regular walking program, you can set the clock back.

Typically, the way an older exerciser should structure a walking program differs little from that of a younger exerciser. Your fitness level should improve at roughly the same rate as your younger counterparts', although you may not be able to cover the same distances as quickly. If you have been extremely sedentary for a long time and have lost your ability to walk with confidence, consider seeking the guidance of a physical therapist — or a personal trainer who is educated and experienced in working with seniors — to help reeducate your walking patterns. Many of my older clients start out walking with the aid of a cane or walker to steady themselves as they gain strength and stamina.

Balancing act

According to statistics reported in the *Journal of the American Geriatric Society,* one out of every three people over the age of 65 falls at least once a year, and about 50 percent of those who break their hips never again gain full walking ability. Many experts believe that age-related trips and falls are associated with a reduced sense of balance and a loss of ability to judge body placement.

Decreased balance due to age is influenced by a number of factors. Special receptor cells located in the skin, muscles, joints, and tendons called *proprioceptors* process information about the body's orientation as it moves through space. As a person gets older, proprioceptors dwindle in sensitivity and give the brain less information and feedback to work with. Slower reflexes and decreased muscular strength, combined with loss of eyesight and depth perception, also contribute to a diminished sense of equilibrium. Flexibility is a factor, too. Lack of flexibility means that you cannot lift your leg as high, as far, or as easily as you used to. This results in a shuffling gait, which in turn makes you more susceptible to literally tripping over your own feet.

Walking helps preserve and restore balance because it requires balance. By comparison, riding a stationary bike does not require much balance, so that form of exercise doesn't help a person with balance problems improve his or her function or mobility in the real world. Balance, like any other skill, requires you to constantly practice to preserve it. Older people who have been sedentary for years often have to relearn the skill of balance while walking in order to remain confidently upright.

Evidence suggests that older adults who include in their fitness regimen exercises (besides walking) that are geared toward improving their sense of balance can reduce the chances of falling. A 1996 study performed at the Department of Neurology at the University of Connecticut School of Medicine in Hartford observed 110 men and women with a mean age of 80. After 3 months of regularly performing moves aimed at sharpening balance, the vast majority of subjects restored their levels of body control and "postural stability" to levels analogous to individuals 3 to 10 years younger.

For example, the following list describes three exercises that may help you improve your balance. If you have balance issues, you may find them difficult to do at first, but with proper training and supervision, most people can master these moves in just a few sessions. After a while, these exercises awaken reflexes and increase body awareness and control on a subconscious level, which can translate into lasting improvements in posture and overall quality of movement.

- ✔ **Walking across a low wooden beam:** This exercise requires a constant correction of knee, hip, and head alignment. All the muscles from head to toe must work properly and in synch in order for you to glide across the beam without extending your arms high in the air or wandering off the edge.

- ✔ **The fulcrum:** With your arms relaxed at your sides, stand on one foot with the other leg held behind you and a few inches off the floor. Lean forward and maintain your balance for up to one minute.

- ✔ **Ball crunch:** Crunches work your abdominal muscles. Lie across a large ball with your feet placed hip-width apart. Place your hands behind your head without clasping your fingers together. Exhale and curl your head, neck, and shoulders up off the ball. Hold a moment. Inhale as you slowly lower to the start. Repeat 8 to 15 times. Do abdominal crunches while attempting to keep the ball as still as possible.

Start out slowly, doing no more than 10 minutes of balance work, two to three times a week. This type of training is deceptively challenging and can leave you feeling exhausted and sore if you overdo it.

Starting from Scratch

For those who are extremely overweight or who have been completely sedentary for years, even a lifestyle walking program similar to the one I describe in Chapter 7 may seem overwhelming. For many reasons, the 20 minutes, three times a week recommended as the minimum amount of exercise by the American College of Sports Medicine may be beyond your ability at the moment.

Starting a walking program from the bottom can be extremely discouraging. I worked with a woman for several years who came to me when she was at least 100 pounds overweight. For years, she barely moved around during the course of her average day, let alone exercised. I remember that during our first session she was so upset about facing the kind of shape she was in that she cried. We started out by exercising while sitting in a chair. I had her lift her legs and move her arms for 30 seconds at a time, and she'd get so out of breath that she'd have to take a break for several minutes. I know she felt discouraged, but she never gave up. Gradually, she was able to move for

10 minutes straight, and eventually we were able to do some marching in place and some walks up and down her hallway. By the time I finished up with her, she had lost about 25 pounds and was well on her way to enjoying a fit and healthy lifestyle. I always considered her an incredibly brave woman.

The important thing to remember when you're starting from rock bottom is *to start.* Everyone has to begin at his or her own starting point, no matter how basic that is. (If you need help starting out, turn to Chapter 2 for some advice on goal setting.) There is no reason to get discouraged or feel bad about yourself, because just embarking on an exercise program is a victory.

Remember, even if a conventional walking program is out of your reach at the moment, it is a good ultimate goal to work toward because it is almost always an attainable aspiration. Going forward, walking is an ideal exercise because, although it is low impact and easy on your body, it also gets results. However, if you have a specific condition, such as heart disease, diabetes, or cancer, I strongly suggest checking in with your doctor for specific exercise instructions. For those starting at a very low level of fitness, I can offer you the following tips:

- ✔ **Do what you can and don't overdo it.** If that means walking for 2 minutes and then taking a rest for 5 minutes, that's fine. Breaking your exercise up into four or five mini-sessions throughout the day may help. It can definitely help you to keep up your efforts on a daily basis.

- ✔ **If walking outdoors or on a treadmill is too strenuous to keep up for more than a few minutes, try walking around your house.** Staying in the house makes it easier to take breaks. For example, you can make it your goal to walk the length of a short hallway several times a day. Or you can walk from the kitchen to the living room, where you can sit down and take a break.

- ✔ **If walking forward is too challenging for the moment, try marching in place with your hand on a chair or some other sturdy object for support.** If standing and moving is too much for you, exercise while sitting in a chair by moving your legs up and down and waving your arms. If need be, start with just a few seconds of exercise at a time and gradually build from there.

- ✔ **Set up a series of short-term goals and focus on those for a while instead of looking toward the long term.** This will keep you from feeling overwhelmed and discouraged. You may not want to take measurements like body fat percentage, body weight, or circumference measurements at first if they discourage or depress you.

- ✔ **Keep a diet and exercise log and review it regularly** so that you can bask in your successes and avoid repeating your mistakes.

- ✔ **Make exercise fun!** Put on some music or exercise with a trusted friend. Do whatever you need to do in order to make exercise a pleasant experience and something you look forward to rather than something you dread.

Exercising with asthma

Medical experts believe that exercise-induced asthma — troubled breathing during exercise — is often exacerbated by cool, dry air. If you are prone to asthma attacks during exercise, try the following suggestions:

✔ Let your doctor know that you want to begin an exercise program. He or she may prescribe a medication strategy to help prevent asthma attacks.

✔ Prevent attacks by pretreatment with prescribed medication.

✔ Warm up slowly and thoroughly.

✔ Go for exercise of long duration and low intensity rather than fast and furious exercise.

✔ Try alternating short spurts of exercise with periods of rest. For instance, walk briskly for 5 minutes and then walk lightly for 5 minutes.

✔ Always carry your inhaler or other medication with you when you exercise.

✔ If you have serious asthma, don't exercise alone. Go to a gym or exercise with a friend. If you walk in a gym, make the staff aware of your condition and the procedures they may need to follow should you have a severe asthma attack while exercising.

✔ Consider using swimming as a cross-training activity. The warm, humid air above the water's surface may help reduce the frequency and severity of asthma attacks.

✔ **Reward yourself.** When you reach a goal, buy yourself that sports watch you've had your eye on or step into a relaxing bubble bath. Avoid rewarding yourself with food as it will only negate your hard-earned calorie burn.

✔ **Don't compare yourself, your program, or your progress to anyone else.**

✔ **Seek the guidance of your physician before beginning an exercise program.** You may also want to consider hiring a personal trainer to help structure your program. If you are mobile enough, you may want to consider joining a support group.

Keeping Fido Fit

My husband often points out to me that dogs are not human and, therefore, technically speaking, should not be considered a "special" population. However, I beg to differ. There are roughly 49 million dogs in this country and over 60 million walkers. My guess is that at least some of those walkers like to walk with their dogs.

My dog, Zoomer, is my best walking buddy. Sometimes I have to beg a friend or family member to go for a walk with me. Not Zoomer. Just the sound of the word "walk" sends him into spasms of delight. Zoomer is a 90-pound, 6-foot long, retired greyhound. Besides being a willing walker, he keeps a close eye on his surroundings, so I feel safe when I walk around the streets and jogging paths of New York City.

A dog can truly be a walker's best friend. Though some breeds are more athletic than others, there's no breed of dog that doesn't make a good walking buddy. I know one woman who proudly struts around with her 2-pound Chihuahua and another woman who takes her two Great Danes for a long stroll each evening and morning. Wherever I go, I see walkers of all shapes and sizes attached by leash to every conceivable type of mutt, mongrel, and purebred.

Dogs, like humans, need to ease into an exercise program, so don't start your pup out on a 10-mile uphill jaunt in the hottest of hot weather. Like you, he needs time to build up his stamina and fitness. Unfortunately, he can't simply tell you he's getting tired and needs a rest, so you have to be careful to look for the signs. If your dog is lagging along behind, panting heavily, or walking with an abnormal gait, that behavior definitely indicates that your four-legged friend is pooped or at least needs to take a break. If he needs to lose weight, manage the process carefully. Allow him to drop his extra puppy fat gradually instead of putting him on a crash diet or exercise program.

Dr. Leigh Semilof, an upstate New York veterinarian I go to for advice about my dog, suggests starting your dog out with 20- to 30-minute walks three to five times a week. After she's established a baseline of fitness — typically 4 to 6 weeks, depending on how out of shape she is to begin with — gradually increase her walking speed, distance, or both.

Assuming your dog is at his ideal weight, up his rations as his mileage and intensity increase. You don't have to fill his bowl to overflowing — a few extra kibbles, a cup of rice, or a couple of doggie treats during the day should satisfy his extra energy needs. You may see a lot of fancy, very expensive dog foods out on the market designed for active dogs. Dr. Semilof says that you don't need to invest in one of these unless your dog is doing an unusually large amount of strenuous activity. Because my dog is extremely active, I feed him Purina Hi Pro Dog Chow. It's formulated for active dogs but costs about a quarter of the price of some of the designer dog foods we tried, and you can buy it in the supermarket. Besides, Zoomer likes it. You may have to experiment with a few foods before you find the one that agrees with your dog's taste buds and your pocketbook.

Keeping your dog cool when you walk

During summer months, exercise your dog before sunup or after sundown to avoid pad blistering and other heat-related conditions. You may want to ice your dog's paws down after a walk if hot pavement is simply unavoidable. On very hot and humid days, let her sit one out in the comfort of air conditioning. She may not be too pleased with you, but it's for her own good.

If you must walk with your dog during daylight hours, stick to the shady routes. Dogs are susceptible to sunburn, especially shorthaired breeds and light-colored dogs, so slather sunscreen on the tip of his nose, over his tummy, and on any other place where he doesn't have an abundance of fur. My dog has no hair on his buttocks as a result of mistreatment when he was a racer, so I have to slather sunscreen on this delicate area before we head out the door; otherwise, he gets as pink as a rare steak. By the way, insect repellent is also a good idea, especially if you go hiking or live in a mosquito-ridden area.

Dogs have no sweat glands, so they don't get soaked like we humans when they exercise. Their version of sweating is panting, and they lose a lot of moisture this way, so you need to keep them properly hydrated during exercise. Carry a water bottle and a cup and offer your dog a drink every 15 minutes or so. When Zoomer and I go hiking, I sometimes carry a collapsible bowl for him like the kind you find in camping supply stores. I also let him splash around in every stream we come to in order to cool his body temperature.

Dehydration and overexposure to the sun can lead to heatstroke, which for dogs as well as humans can be deadly. Watch for symptoms of this condition, including uncontrollable panting and frothing at the mouth. If you note these symptoms, call your vet immediately.

Walking your dog in cold weather

For the most part, a dog's fur can protect him against extreme cold. For this reason, it's not a good idea to clip your dog or bathe him during cold weather months. Short-haired dogs or dogs that don't carry a lot of body fat should wear a coat or a sweater whenever the thermometer dips below the freezing point. You may think that a sweater makes your dog look silly. I know I think that my dog looks ridiculous in his cape, but I also know that it's absolutely necessary to protect him from frostbite. If you believe that your dog needs a more macho look, try fitting him with an old sweatshirt.

I order my dog's coats through a catalog called *Animal Magnetism*. It carries a good selection of unusual items and sizes for many different breeds, but especially hounds.

Unless you are traveling over familiar territory, don't let your dog off the leash in the snow. Dogs can lose their scent in the snow and get lost. Many dogs are also frightened and confused by heavy snowfall. It's also harder for your dog to walk in snow because she sinks down and has to work a lot harder to move forward. Take this into consideration and adjust your mileage accordingly.

In general, the area of most concern during the winter months are your dog's paws. When you come indoors, check for ice balls that form in between her toes. Salt and other harsh chemicals may cause irritation, too. Wiping her paws with a warm, wet cloth usually takes care of these problems. Many pet stores sell special paw wax or dog shoes to protect canine feet from the elements. Personally, I can't bring myself to buy shoes for my dog.

Other tips for walking with your dog

Here are some more tips to make exercising with your four-legged friend an enjoyable experience for both of you:

- Precede each workout with a 5- to 10-minute walk to let him relieve himself and mark his territory.

- Obey all leash laws.

- Carry a scooper or bags to clean up all messes.

- Don't allow your dog to mangle flower beds or otherwise damage property. Don't allow her to chase other dogs or animals or disturb other walkers' enjoyment.

- If your dog tries to stop during your walk, give a firm but gentle tug on the leash. After a while, he'll bypass all but the most irresistible sights and scents. If he absolutely must stop to check something out, cut him some slack.

- When walking on or along the side of a road, walk facing traffic and train your dog to stay on your left side so as not to interfere with traffic flow.

- Teach her the "heel" command as well as other obedience basics so that she doesn't charge across busy intersections or drag you around as you walk.

Finally, when you're not sure what's best for your dog's safety or health, ask your veterinarian. You can also check out *Dogs For Dummies* by Gina Spadafori (IDG Books Worldwide, Inc.).

Chapter 15

A Pain in the . . .

. . . .

In This Chapter

▶ Preventing blisters

▶ Coping with corns and bunions

▶ Nursing neuromas and plantar fasciitis

▶ Relieving shin splints

▶ Standing up to low back pain

▶ Picking yourself up after an "oops injury"

. . . .

*W*alkers encounter fewer injuries than just about any other group of fitness enthusiasts. In fact, many people turn to walking after racking up their share of injuries from other activities. Runners with knee problems are common walking converts as are inline skaters who've taken one spill too many.

That's not to say walkers never feel an ache or a pain. Everyone gets a little twinge every now and then. When you first begin a walking routine, for instance, you should expect your muscles to feel a little sore and stiff. That's what walkers call "good" pain, the kind of pain that's a natural extension of increasing your activity and waking up dormant muscles. Muscle soreness usually goes away by the end of your first week of regular exercise.

In this chapter, I review the "bad" pain that accompanies the most prevalent walking injuries as well as strategies for prevention and treatment. Fortunately, most of the physical ailments that result from walking are easily treatable and rarely set you back more than a few days.

Blisters

Blisters are caused by friction and irritation, usually from something that rubs against your foot. Some walkers are more prone to blistering than others, but everyone is more susceptible during hot or wet weather. Some of my clients tell me that they tend to develop blisters during seasonal changes when temperatures vary widely from day to day.

You'd never think something as small as a blister would be so painful and debilitating, but I can tell you from experience, it is. I remember a hike I did one particularly hot day. About an hour into the walk, I realized that the new shoes that I was wearing had several prominent seams that rubbed against the bottom and sides of my foot. By the time I completed the hike, I was in so much pain that I was hobbling around as if my ankles were tied together. When I removed my shoes, a wall of blisters surrounded the outer edges and the bottoms of my feet. It was several days before I could walk comfortably again.

The best way to prevent blisters is to avoid them in the first place. If you're thin-skinned or live in a warm or rainy climate, you may never be able to completely blister-proof your feet, but taking precautions can minimize the severity and frequency. Blister prevention includes three strategic factors: proper shoes, socks, and lubrication.

Wear shoes that fit

When your shoes are too big, your feet slide around from side to side as you walk, and that may cause blisters. On the other hand, if your shoes are too small, they can rub against your feet and create hot spots and, ultimately, blisters. Ill-fitting shoes do the most damage when you go up and down hills because your feet jam up against the toe box and heel of your shoes, creating blisters on the tips and crevices of your toes.

I know that many people buy walking and other types of shoes that don't quite fit right in the hopes that they can break in the shoes over time. This is a mistake. Shoes should feel comfortable from the instant you take your first step in them and until the moment you replace them. They shouldn't require any stretching, padding, or taping to make them wearable.

A properly fitting shoe should have the same basic shape as your foot: The shoe should be wide where your foot is wide and narrow where your foot is narrow. It should also be flexible enough so that it bends and flexes as your foot moves through your walking stride. There should be about a thumbnail's width between your longest toe and the front of the shoe, and when you lace the shoe up, your foot should be held firmly in place without feeling like it's in a straitjacket.

Try on shoes at the end of the day when your feet are their largest because of swelling. It's not enough to just stick the shoes on your feet. Always walk a few brisk circles around the perimeter of the store or the length of the mall to see whether they feel right when you're in motion. Besides fit, be on the look-out for prominent, ragged stitching or seams — big-time blister-causing culprits. Who hasn't had the back of their heels rubbed bloody by poor-quality stitching? (For more shoe-buying tips, see Chapter 3.)

Wear socks

I had a client who insisted on walking, cycling, and running sans socks but couldn't understand why his heels and the tops of his feet were always riddled with blisters. (His shoes smelled, too.) Socks provide a protective layer between your foot and your shoe. Without them, your feet are subject to incredible friction.

The socks you wear should conform perfectly to your feet and should have no wrinkles, bunching, or extra folds. Natural fibers like cotton and wool feel, well, more natural. But when they get wet, they lose their shape and take a long time to dry. Socks made from synthetics like nylon dry quickly and hold their shape, but they may be abrasive.

You need to experiment to see what works best for you. I've had good luck with socks made from CoolMax, a thin material designed to wick away moisture and hold its shape even when wet. I recommend buying brand-name socks rather than the six-pack of athletic socks found in discount stores. High-quality socks are way more expensive but cause fewer problems in the long run.

Some people claim that wearing two pairs of socks helps prevent blisters because they rub against each other instead of your foot. But if both pairs don't fit to a tee and line up exactly, this strategy can backfire. One of my clients suggests something that I'm not sure men may go for but does seem to work: Wear a pair of knee-high stockings underneath your socks. The socks slip against the nylon while the nylon remains conformed to your feet no matter what. I have successfully experimented with this technique — but I think the stockings feel strange.

Lubricate

If you're seriously blister prone, try lubing up your feet with petroleum jelly. Make sure that you coat your foot thoroughly, especially at the back of the heel and in between your toes. Even though the slippery, oily feeling takes some getting used to, "gooping up" has never failed me. If this is just too icky for you to deal with, try sprinkling talcum powder in your socks and shoes. I personally don't find powder as effective, but it's certainly neater.

Blister remedies: If, in spite of your best efforts, you develop blisters anyway, leave them alone as long as they don't interfere with your walking routine. If they balloon up to the point where they cause pain, try padding them with moleskin or bandages. If that doesn't help, drain them by cutting a small incision with a sterile razor blade or nail scissors. (To sterilize, boil the scissors in water for 15 minutes and then wipe them clean with rubbing alcohol.) Clean the infected area with an antiseptic and then bandage.

I usually paint my blisters with a liquid bandage; these products protect and toughen up the area, thereby helping to prevent future blister uprisings.

If you have recurring hot spots that seem to blister up no matter what you do, get an old pair of shoes and cut a hole in the corresponding area so that the offending spot has nothing to rub against. This should eliminate painful friction and allow the blister a chance to heal completely. In the meantime, toughen up the area by painting it frequently with a liquid bandage.

Corns and Bunions

Corns and bunions, those bumps and knobbies that crop up all over your feet, especially on the sides, tops, and crevices of your toes, are caused by shoes that are too tight. Often, your walking shoes aren't the culprit; it's those pointy, narrow shoes that you wear to work. In cultures where shoe wearing isn't common, feet riddled with corns and bunions are nonexistent.

Corn and bunion remedies: Get rid of offending shoes and you can greatly reduce — and even eliminate — the problem. Store-bought pads, doughnuts, and moleskin work to a point, as does the cutting-an-opening-in-the-shoe trick I mention in the "Blisters" section of this chapter.

Give your corns a few strokes with an emery board each day to decrease their surface area and to restore some flexibility to the skin. Keep a pumice stone in the shower for the same purpose.

If your corns and bunions get so large that it becomes impossible to find comfortable shoes, go to a podiatrist for professional treatment.

I don't recommend buying over-the-counter remedies for corn and bunion removal, especially those that contain salicylic acid as the active ingredient. My friend and podiatrist, Dr. Lou Galli, says that these aren't very effective and may make matters worse by ulcerating the skin. And no matter what, do not — repeat do not — attempt to cut the bumps down with a razor blade or knife! Dr. Lou says you'd be surprised how many people are brave enough (and foolish enough) to attempt this. Doing so is like begging for an infection.

Neuromas

My first experience with a neuroma was years ago when my client Vivian complained of pain in her two middle toes closest to her pinkie toe, a pain she described as a strong electrical shock shooting up through the ball of her foot out through the end of her toes. I sent her to New York's foot guru, Dr. Lou Galli, and she came back with a diagnosis of Morton's neuroma.

A neuroma is a bundle of exposed or inflamed nerve endings, usually located on the lower part of the two toes closest to the pinkie toe, but you can develop them in other toes as well. There's no swelling, and you may feel pain at times other than when you're walking, even when your feet are up and not bearing any body weight.

The cause? Here again, tight shoes may be the problem. The tighter the shoe, the more pressure on the nerves of the feet. Pounding on hard surfaces like cement or asphalt, especially if you're overweight, if you tend to slam your foot down as you walk, or if you spend too much time on your toes, can also be a contributing factor. Then again, sometimes there's no apparent reason at all for this pesky injury — some people just get them. Vivian, for instance, is a small woman who is careful about the shoes she wears and almost always walks on a treadmill.

Neuroma remedy: Your first go-to remedy for a neuroma flare-up is ice.

I like to fill a Dixie cup with water and stick it in the freezer. After the water freezes, you can peel down the top portion of the cup to form a snow cone of sorts, which you can use to rub all over the affected area. Moving the ice helps the cold penetrate deeper and covers more surface area.

Placing padding directly behind a neuroma may help ease the pressure. Use surgical padding found in good medical drugstores, or foam rubber held in place with athletic tape. I know some people who glue their padding directly into the insides of their shoes so that they don't have to tape their feet before every walk.

If a neuroma becomes a recurring problem, don't ignore it. Get thee to a podiatrist. A podiatrist may make you a special shoe insert to minimize the pain, or he may inject cortisone. As a last resort, you can have neuromas removed surgically.

Plantar Fasciitis

Have you ever felt pain in the bottoms of your feet first thing in the morning that seems to get better as the day wears on? This is very likely plantar fasciitis, an inflammation of the tough fibrous band of tissue that runs the length of the bottom of your foot. You may feel the pain after you walk but not necessarily when you walk. Those first ten steps from the bedroom to the bathroom each morning are usually the most uncomfortable.

Many activities can cause plantar fasciitis: over-training, misalignment of the foot, walking on hard surfaces, doing a lot of hill or speed training, and generally stressing tight hamstring and calf muscles. And of course, there's the by now familiar culprit — ill-fitting shoes.

So the first thing you can do, even before your arches feel strained or pained, is check your shoes. Is there enough bend at the ball of the foot? Are they wide enough? Are they flexible and not overly built up through the arch? Switch your shoes if the answer to any of these questions is no.

Another way to prevent fasciitis and a host of other maladies is to keep your hamstrings and calf muscles loose and flexible. See Chapter 12 for stretching information. If you're prone to fasciitis flare-ups, stay off hard surfaces whenever possible, avoid hills, and cross-train with non-weight-bearing activities like cycling and swimming.

Plantar fasciitis remedies: This injury responds well to ice and elevation. Ice your feet immediately after walking for 10 to 20 minutes. Use the ice cup method I describe under the "Neuromas" section or, if you can stand it, plunge your feet into a bucket of ice water. When you're done icing, prop your feet up for a few minutes. Foot massage may offer some additional relief, especially if you can get someone else to do it.

A physician may recommend taking an over-the-counter anti-inflammatory medication such as aspirin to reduce swelling, but don't self-medicate, especially if you have allergies or other medical conditions.

Over-the-counter arch supports and heel cups may help you in the short term, but inevitably you're going to have to seek a more permanent solution, such as podiatrist-designed and -fitted inserts called orthotics; these correct weight distribution along the foot.

Shin Splints

Sooner or later, every walker develops a case of shin splints, the catchall term for shin pain. You may get them from walking longer or faster than usual, or from walking on a dirt road when you usually walk on pavement — or vice versa. New shoes, hill work, and muscular imbalances can all lead to a case of the shin splint blues. And sometimes they may crop up for seemingly no reason at all.

Shin splints are a pain in the lower leg due to inflammation of the muscles or tendons. For various reasons, your lower leg bones brace themselves to antici-pate the jolt from the next step. This stress leads to swelling, tearing, and inflammation of the surrounding muscles.

To avoid shin splints, strengthen your shin muscles so that they are in balance with your calf muscles. (See Chapter 11 for some shin strengthening suggestions.) Replace your walking shoes often so that your shins don't take a pounding from lack of cushioning. Make sure that your shoes fit properly. If a shoe is too large or too wide, your toes clutch the bottom of the shoe, thereby causing strain to those front lower leg muscles and increasing the frequency and severity of shin splint episodes.

Shin splint remedies: Ice helps by reducing inflammation and by dulling the pain. Some people find that wrapping heating pads or warm washcloths around their shins offers some relief.

Cut back on your mileage or switch to a non-weight-bearing activity until the pain completely disappears. Replace your shoes every 1,000 miles or more frequently if you're prone to shin splints.

 Whatever you do, don't ignore chronic or extreme shin splints. Have them checked out by a good orthopedist or other trusted medical professional. Left untreated, they can develop into more serious problems such as large muscle tears and full-blown stress fractures.

Lower Back Pain

Back pain is another one of those catchall terms for a problem that manifests itself in many ways for many reasons. However, most walkers who experience back pain do so because of poor walking posture. Walking with your upper body forward or rounded is one of the quickest paths to an achy back. Weak and/or tight hamstring, hip, or abdominal muscles are often part of the problem. When your muscles are out of balance, your whole stride and body posture are thrown off-balance, too.

To prevent back pain when you feel it coming on, review your walking posture checklists from Chapters 7 through 10. Slow down your pace or walk on a treadmill for a few days so that you can really zero in on form. Keep your muscles strong by doing the exercises mentioned in Chapter 11. Stretch your muscles by doing the exercises outlined in Chapter 12.

Lower back pain remedies: If you're having a lower back pain episode, a warm bath or moist heat are probably your best bet. Ice is also an option but only if you don't tense up your lower back when it's applied.

For low back pain that isn't too debilitating, some gentle stretching can help loosen you up. Some of my clients rely on a chiropractor for their back problems, but I've never gone to one myself, so I can't claim firsthand experience. Ditto for acupuncture. (I've heard good things about such treatments.) My husband, who is prone to back pain during times of stress, swears by massage. Physical therapy is also a common treatment, and it's usually covered by insurance as long as it's prescribed by a physician.

You may have to try a few treatments and strategies before you hit on one that works best for you. In rare instances, your physician may recommend back surgery to correct a chronic, severe back problem, but many experts now conclude that surgery is not helpful and may cause more problems than it solves.

Oops Injuries

An "oops injury" is my phrase for any injury that's a result of clumsiness, carelessness, or plain bad luck. When you step off a curb the wrong way and twist your ankle, that's an oops injury. When you trip over your own feet for no apparent reason, that's an oops injury. I'm always surprised at how many people hurt themselves in this way while out for a walk. On the other hand, I'm the charter member of the oops injury club.

One time I was walking along, lost in my own thoughts, and I walked smack into a stop sign, severely bruising both my forehead and my ego.

The best prevention for an oops injury is paying attention. It's nice to let yourself relax and think about other things, but keep at least one corner of your mind on your surroundings. I have one client who was so out of touch with reality that he walked off a bridge. Luckily, a stream broke his fall.

Oops injury remedies: Most oops injuries can be treated with ice or an adhesive bandage. Sometimes, if you've done a real number, they require a trip to the doctor or the emergency room. Make an honest assessment based on the amount of pain, swelling, or bleeding that's present. You may be reluctant to seek medical treatment if you've hurt yourself in a really dumb or embarrassing way, but when in doubt, swallow your pride and make the trip — better a little embarrassment than a fractured ankle or a broken toe.

Chapter 16

The Complete Treadmill Guide

According to the Sporting Goods Manufacturers Association, an organization that tracks trends in fitness and exercise, nearly 33 million people work out on a treadmill on a regular basis. The treadmill is the only aerobic exercise machine that has grown in usage every year since 1986; in fact, usage has increased a whopping 648 percent over the past ten years.

I see evidence of this treadmill trend whenever I walk into any of the fitness centers I manage during the prime-time busy hours. I can virtually guarantee that, even if every other piece of aerobic equipment is vacant, the treadmills will be doing a brisk business. I'm sure that this is true of almost every gym in America.

Treadmills are especially popular in crowded, polluted cities, where a walk outdoors isn't always practical or safe. They also get used more on days when it's too hot or too cold to venture a walk outside. We walkers like working out on a treadmill because we don't require any extra skills to use them.

Because treadmills are so popular these days, I devote this entire chapter to the machine that allows you to "walk nowhere fast." I describe common treadmill features and how to use them, provide an overview of the best treadmill training techniques, and give you the scoop on how to purchase a treadmill of your own.

Walking on a Belt Versus a Beltway

Walking on a treadmill may seem like the equivalent of walking in place because you don't go anywhere, but physiologically and mechanically, it isn't that much different from walking outdoors. Some studies do show that you may burn fewer calories and use fewer muscles for any given speed on a treadmill. However, as long as you walk at the same intensity and reach the same heart rate as you do when you walk outdoors, the differences are inconsequential.

Today's treadmills are springier and more shock-absorbing than ever, so most people find that walking on one is kinder to their joints than hard surfaces like concrete and asphalt. Treadmills are also easier on the knees and ankles than running tracks. Even if a track is outfitted with a special rubberized surface, walking in circles forces the inside leg to work harder than the outside leg, which can lead to muscle imbalances and overuse injuries.

My friend Laura used to walk the heavily banked path around the perimeter of Prospect Park in Brooklyn until her knees began to ache all the time. The slant in the road placed one leg higher than the other, and over time, this awkward form threw her gait and walking form out of whack. This is a fairly common problem for people who walk a lot on slanted or uneven surfaces. Switching to a treadmill for a few weeks took care of the problem for Laura.

If you're recovering from any sort of injury, it's not a bad idea to start walking on a treadmill first before you head outdoors to walk.

Now for the downside of treadmill walking: It can be mind-numbingly boring. The scenery never changes, and there's little to occupy your mind. For this reason, you probably need to get out and see the world every once in a while instead of walking on the treadmill every single day. Treadmill workouts are most effective and interesting when they have a purpose and a definite structure. Later in this chapter, I suggest some purposeful and structured workouts and give you several strategies for beating treadmill boredom.

Buying a Treadmill

If you're thinking about buying a treadmill, you're not alone. In the U.S. alone, more than $960 million was spent on treadmills in 1995 (the last year statistics were available), up 12 percent from the year before. But, before you drop a few thousand on your dream machine, you should know that not all treadmills are created equal.

Knowing which kind of treadmill to buy

Treadmills come in two basic versions: motorless and motorized. Which one should you buy?

Treadmills, unplugged

Though they cost only a couple hundred dollars, non-motorized treadmills, which require you to push the walking belt along with your feet, are not a good choice. It's nearly impossible to get the belt moving unless you incline the machine. In addition, at faster walking speeds, the belt tends to catch and stick at irregular intervals, causing you to stutter-step along. If you weigh less than 150 pounds, you will find it nearly impossible to keep the belt moving for any length of time unless you are on an extreme incline.

I keep looking for a non-motorized treadmill that works properly, but I haven't found one yet, even though I've tried dozens. Although they're budget friendly, I think you will be sorely disappointed in the workout they deliver, so I'm against spending any amount of money on a non-motorized treadmill.

Treadmills with motors

Treadmills that use a motor to power the walking belt move at a smooth, consistent speed that you can vary with the touch of a button. Even though you'll have to spend between $1,000 and $5,000 for a motorized treadmill, this is definitely the way to go.

Unfortunately, I can't in good conscience recommend any bargain-priced treadmills. Inexpensive discount and department store models, fold-up treadmills, and machines with arm poles are generally poorly designed and cheaply made. Although they cost only a few hundred dollars, they're wobbly and won't hold up even with light use. After they break, you're out of luck; these stores don't have service departments to fix them. Stick with high-quality manufacturers and buy only from sporting good stores that specialize in selling exercise equipment.

Good treadmills include Trotter, Star Trac, Landice, True, and Precor. Those brands sell models that fall within the $1,500 to $5,000 range. The best brand I've found for under $1,000 is Icon, but I don't recommend it if you're very heavy, you walk very fast, or you tend to slam your feet down when you walk. My favorite brand is Trotter. I have my trusty Trotter tucked behind my couch and use it a couple times a week.

Here are the must-have features to look for when you're purchasing a treadmill of your own:

✔ **Speed and elevation controls:** High-quality treadmills move at speeds ranging from 1 to 10 mph and have a motor rating of at least 1.5 *continuous-duty* horsepower. (The meaningless term *peak duty* is tossed around by a lot of salespeople. It refers to how hard the machine can work for an instance rather than how well it will perform over a long, *continuous* period of time.) The better treadmills also can be elevated by pressing a button rather than using a manual crank.

✔ **Safety features:** An emergency stop button and an automatic slow-start speed of 1 mph or less are a must. A front handrail is also helpful for maintaining balance and is safer than side rails, which may actually disrupt your balance if they impede your arm swing.

Consider a machine that requires a security code or special magnet to start it, especially if you have young children. If you stumble, the magnet breaks contact, and the belt quickly comes to a halt so that you don't shoot off the back like a piece of luggage on a conveyor belt. Some treadmills prevent falls with a sonar sensor that monitors your position on the walking surface and automatically adjusts speed and elevation to keep you in the center of the belt.

✔ **Walking belt:** The surface directly underneath the belt, called the deck, should be laminated pressed wood rather than ordinary plywood. On better-quality treadmills, the deck is impregnated with lubricants to reduce friction and wear and tear. Look for a machine with a deck that can be rotated when it begins to wear down; this feature can more than double the life span of the machine. (Ask your salesperson whether the deck on a treadmill can be rotated; you can't tell just by looking at the treadmill.)

To reduce impact on your joints, most manufacturers insert rubber disks, springs, or some other shock-absorbing device underneath the deck. Although this is a joint-saving idea to be sure, be careful when checking out this feature. Just as with beds and office chairs, an overly soft surface may actually contribute to joint problems. You should feel like you're floating along with a little extra spring in your step, not like you're bounding along on a trampoline.

✔ **Extra features:** At the very least, you'll probably want a control panel with a readout that gives you information on speed, pace, elapsed time, calories burned, and calories burned per hour. Fancy features like a heart rate monitor and built-in programs can be very engaging, but they quickly pump up the price. If you don't care about bells and whistles, you can save big bucks by sticking with a no-frills model that has your basic safety features and gives you your time, speed, and distance.

Exercising caution before you buy

Before you set foot in a treadmill dealer's store, measure the space where you plan to put your treadmill and be sure that it fits through the door into the room. Check out ceiling height, too: You don't want to raise the incline only to have your head poke through a ceiling tile.

Nothing less than a one-year on-site warranty is acceptable. Also make sure that someone within 300 miles will honor the warranty.

Trotter treadmills have an exceptional three-year warranty, and Star Trac boasts its own service network. Ask about sales or discounts for floor models and price breaks on delivery and installation.

In general, I don't recommend buying a used treadmill at a garage sale or auction unless you know how to fix it yourself. The Gym Source, an exercise equipment dealer in the northeastern part of the U.S., sells refurbished tread-mills and honors the full warranties. If you can find a deal like that, go for it. You'll probably save a lot of money.

Here is perhaps the most important advice I can give you on buying a treadmill: Take a test drive on several machines so that you get a good comparison of their feel and features. After all, the one you like best is the one you'll use the most.

Reading the Readout

When you first look at the information panel of a treadmill, it may seem as complicated as the control panel of a DC-10 jet. I've seen people take a look at all the buttons, numbers, and flashing lights of one of the more complicated treadmill panels, shrug their shoulders, and walk away.

Becoming familiar with the information panel on your treadmill is as impor-tant as tying your walking shoes properly. The average treadmill provides much useful feedback. Knowing how to interpret all those buttons, numbers, and flashing lights helps you to get more out of your workout.

Here's a rundown on some of the common treadmill panel features, what they mean, and how to use the feedback they provide. Not every treadmill you meet has all these features, but many of them do.

✔ **Start button:** The start button obviously starts the walking belt moving. Most newer treadmills automatically start at a very slow speed, usually around 1 mph. In other words, even if the last person to use it was jet-ting along at 10 mph and suddenly stopped the belt, the next time it starts up, it will automatically default to a crawl pace. Believe it or not, this feature is a relatively new development. Someone flying off the treadmill as a result of an unexpected quick start was a daily occurrence when I first started working in health clubs.

Some treadmills require you to enter a special code or press a combination of keys to start the belt. This feature, available primarily on home models, is invaluable, especially if you have children.

As if matters aren't complicated enough, some treadmills have two start buttons: The main start button, which is usually red or green, starts the belt moving. The second start button starts the timer and odometer.

✔ **Stop button:** Stop buttons are usually labeled "stop" or "end workout." Some models have two stop buttons. One stop button stops the timer and odometer on your workout, while the other (usually a large red button) is an emergency feature that instantly stops the belt.

✔ **Reset, clear, store:** The reset button clears off the stats from the last workout and starts you out at zero time and distance. Sometimes it also resets the belt to a slower speed, so check that out before you press it. The reset function is sometimes labeled "clear." Some treadmills have the option of storing your workout stats or the actual speed, distance, and incline of the program you just completed. You can recall these same options with the touch of a button. If you have a favorite workout, this feature is particularly useful.

✔ **Speedometer and pace-ometer:** Most treadmills give you information on both the pace and speed that you walk. What's the difference?

Speed, which refers to how fast you're walking, is usually measured in miles per hour, just like the speed of a car. Typical walking speeds range from 2 to 4.5 mph. *Pace,* which refers to how long it takes you to cover 1 mile, is usually measured in miles per minute. So if you walk at 15 minutes per mile (or you're doing a 15-minute mile), that means it takes you 15 minutes to cover 1 mile.

One set of buttons increases and decreases walking speed and pace. (When you walk at a faster speed, your pace also increases.) Some treadmills display both speed and pace at once, and some have a "cycle" button that you press to display one piece of information at a time.

Whether you focus on speed or pace is a matter of personal preference. I personally like to know my pace. I feel that knowing how long completing a mile is going to take tells me more about the quality of my workout. When I think of my workout in miles per hour, I can't shake the car analogy out of my head, and there's no way I can favorably compare myself to something that usually moves at 65 mph.

✔ **Elevation or incline:** This feature simulates walking up a hill. Typically, you press a button to raise yourself up or lower yourself down one degree at a time. Most treadmills allow an incline from 0 to 15 percent, though some models incline as high as 25 percent. Incline, by the way, is based upon a relationship to a 90-degree angle, which represents something that is completely vertical (straight up and down). For instance, a 5 percent incline is the equivalent of 5 percent of a 90-degree angle. Here's a way to equate incline on a treadmill to the steepness of hills that you may encounter while walking outdoors: A 5 percent incline is the equivalent of a moderately steep hill, a 10 percent incline is equivalent to a steep hill, and a 15 percent incline is equivalent to a *very* steep hill.

✔ A few treadmills (Precor and Trotter, for example) decline from –1 to –5 percent to simulate walking down a hill. I am in love with this feature, which I use to train my clients who fast walk, race walk, or frequently walk on hilly terrain. Walking downhill uses your muscles *eccentrically*, that is, in a lengthened position. Eccentric training has a tendency to cause extreme muscle soreness. My theory is that downhill training on a treadmill helps build up tolerance to eccentric training and thus helps eliminate muscle soreness after really hard workouts.

✔ **Timer:** Most treadmills usually start a timer running as soon as you turn on the belt. Some treadmills, however, allow you to press a separate button to start the timer. I like having a separate start timer because you get your true walking time. Without this feature, doing accurate time trials is difficult.

✔ **Calorimeter:** The most accurate treadmills ask for your body weight at the beginning of each workout. Because walking involves supporting your body as you move (as opposed to, say, cycling or swimming), you get a more precise reading when you factor body weight into the mathematical formulas that the treadmill uses to estimate calories. If your treadmill does not ask for your weight, it probably automatically bases the calorie readout on the assumption that you weigh 150 pounds. Keep in mind that if you weigh less than that, the calorie readout will be too high, and if you weigh more than, the calorie readout will be too low.

✔ **Programs:** Fancier treadmills have preset programs. You select which one you want to do at the beginning of your workout, and speed and grade automatically change at set intervals. Different programs are geared toward different types of goals. Some are based on speed, others on distance, others on changing inclines. A few treadmills allow you to create and store your own custom workouts.

All treadmills have a manual mode that allows you to create your own workout as you go along. When you press the manual button, *you* control how tough the workout is — you push one arrow to speed up the pace, another to slow down. If your treadmill doesn't have a manual button, all workouts are probably manual.

✔ **Heart rate monitor:** One of the latest developments in treadmills — and exercise equipment in general — is heart rate monitor compatibility. Users of Polar brand heart rate monitors can strap their monitors around their chest. The treadmill then picks up the signal and beams it on to the control panel. For those who use heart rate as an indicator of workout intensity, this feature is very useful indeed. It saves you the trouble of glancing at your heart rate watch every few minutes to check your heart rate, something that's very hard to do when you're moving along.

A few treadmills have special metal bars built into the handrails that read heart rate. You hold on to the bar for 15 seconds or more so that the bar can read your heart rate and send it to the control panel. I don't really like these bars because, by definition, they disrupt your workout by making you hold on for at least 15 seconds. When you hold on, you don't have to work as hard, resulting in a heart rate readout that isn't as accurate as it should be.

✔ **Other features:** Many models use some sort of graph to represent the workout. Trotter treadmills, for instance, chart your progress by using yellow dots to represent speed and green dots to represent incline. As the workout progresses, the dots march across the screen. The dots on Star Trac treadmills travel around a circular 1-mile track.

Preventing Tread Dread

To the uninitiated, walking on a treadmill can seem like the exercise equivalent of Chinese water torture. You can muster up some treadmill motivation in one of two ways: You can either tune into the experience or tune out completely. If you frequently walk on a treadmill, you'll probably tune in on some days and tune out on others.

Tuning in

With all the information that your treadmill gives you the ability to monitor and process, think of yourself as the captain of a big ship embarking on an important journey. Here are some examples of the different kinds of journeys you can take:

Interval training

What it is: Interval training involves alternating periods of high intensity with periods of low intensity. Because interval training can take a lot out of you, I recommend doing it once or twice a week at the most.

The treadmill advantage: Interval training is a great way to increase your fitness level, burn calories, and experiment with working out at higher levels. I love to do interval training on the treadmill. In many ways, it is far more effective than interval training on the road because you always know exactly how far and fast you've been going and for how long — there's no way to fudge it. Many of my clients tell me that they work their intervals harder on a treadmill because they have to set a speed and work against it rather than try to motivate themselves to move their legs faster. (For more about interval training, flip to Chapter 13.)

How to do it: A typical treadmill interval session should last from 30 to 60 minutes total. Always start with a warm-up at any easy pace for 5 to 10 minutes. Then move into the meat of your workout, the interval phase. This is where you alternate a period of fast walking with a period of slower walking. The length and intensity of your work intervals depend upon your fitness level and goals. In general, faster, shorter work intervals, lasting from 30 seconds to 2 minutes, help develop speed and power. They're useful for anyone who is trying to build muscle, training for an athletic event, or doing a lot of hill training. Moderately fast, longer intervals lasting from 2 to 5 minutes burn a lot of fat and calories and help increase overall endurance.

The length of your rest intervals depends mainly on your fitness level. The better shape you're in, the shorter your rest intervals will be. When you first begin interval training, you may want to start with a 1:2 ratio; that is, for every 1 minute of hard work you do, do an easy recovery pace for 2 minutes. Gradually increase that to a 1:1 work/recovery ratio and then a 2:1 work/rest ratio.

After you have completed the desired number of intervals, be sure to finish up with a 5- to 10-minute cool-down and a stretch. The total number of interval cycles you do depends once again on your goals and fitness level. The longer your workout, the more calories you'll burn. However, most walkers find that a 30-minute interval workout, which includes the warm-up and the cool-down, is a good, challenging introductory workout.

How to use the panel: The treadmill panel is a great tool to use for precise interval training. Focus primarily on the timer and speed buttons. A good rule is to pick a warm-up pace that is very comfortable and very easy to maintain. Your first interval should be approximately from 0.5 to 0.7 miles per hour higher than your warm-up pace. You can evaluate from there. Was it too hard? Was it too easy? If a heart rate monitor is available, use it to help deter-mine intensity and adjust accordingly.

Sample workout: I recommend some specific speeds and times for interval training in Table 16-1, but please adjust accordingly to your abilities. Use the speed arrows to change the speed, and keep a sharp eye on the timer so that you make changes at precise intervals. If you're using a heart rate monitor, note your heart rate during each interval and how much it slows down during each recovery interval. Write down as much of this information as possible; you may find it useful to compare workouts that are a couple of months apart to gauge your improvement.

Table 16-1	Sample Treadmill Interval Session	
Workout Segment	*Speed*	*Time*
Warm-up	3.0 mph	5 minutes
Work interval 1	3.5 mph	3 minutes
Rest interval 1	3.0 mph	3 minutes
Work interval 2	3.7 mph	3 minutes
Rest interval 2	3.0 mph	3 minutes
Work interval 3	4.0 mph	1 minute
Rest interval 3	3.0 mph	1 minute
Work interval 4	3.7 mph	2 minutes
Rest interval 4	3.0 mph	2 minutes
Work interval 5	3.5 mph	2 minutes
Cool-down	3.0 mph	5 minutes
Total time		30 minutes

Hill training

What it is: You use the incline feature to manipulate the difficulty of your workout. You can add in hills every day, but do intense hill work only once or twice a week.

The treadmill advantage: Hill work tones the butt and thigh muscles and makes you a stronger overall walker. Hill training on the treadmill allows you to create your own hills, something that's difficult to do when you're training outdoors. For instance, you may not be able to find a moderately steep hill along your walking route that takes you 2 minutes to walk up. On a treadmill, you can whip up any hill you like with the touch of a button.

How to do it: You can set a steady speed and change the intensity of your workout by changing the incline. Or you can use a combination of speeds and grades to achieve the same effects.

I recommend using primarily moderate to steep inclines and using very steep inclines sparingly or staying away from them altogether. Very steep inclines of 15 percent or higher can be hard on your knees and ankles and may cause shin splints or calf spasms. By experimenting with hills of 2 to 12 percent incline that take you from 30 seconds to 5 minutes to climb, you'll get the maximum benefits from hills without a greater risk of injury.

Start each hill workout with a warm-up at an easy pace with no incline and then move into the hilly portion of your workout. Alternate periods of hill walking with periods of rest and then finish up with a cool-down. You can come up with a virtually endless combination of rest-to-hill ratios. In general, if you're a hill neophyte, start out by alternating equal hill intervals with flat intervals to give your shins and calves time to adapt. Most treadmill hill workouts last 30 to 60 minutes, but you can make them shorter or longer depending on your ambition, goals, and time constraints.

How to use the panel: If you're setting one speed and manipulating only the incline, this makes your job easier — all you have to do is manipulate the up and down incline arrows. Note how each change in incline affects your heart rate and workout difficulty. You can see a big difference between walking at 3.5 mph and 0 percent grade and walking at 3.5 mph on a 6 percent grade.

Record your responses at various points throughout the workout so that you can use it to measure improvement. As walking up hills becomes easier, you can make the inclines higher, walk uphill longer, or bump up a combo of speed and incline.

Sample workout: I recommend a set speed of 3.0 mph for the warm-up and cool-down and a workout speed of 3.5 mph (see Table 16-2). Please adjust accordingly to suit your abilities. Use the incline arrows to change the speed, and keep a sharp eye on the timer so that you make the changes at precise intervals.

Table 16-2	Sample Treadmill Hill Training	
Workout Segment	_Incline_	_Time_
Warm-up (3.0 mph)	0 percent	5 minutes
Work interval 1 (3.5 mph)	4 percent	2 minutes
Rest interval 1 (3.5 mph)	0 percent	2 minutes
Work interval 2 (3.5 mph)	6 percent	2 minutes
Rest interval 2 (3.5 mph)	0 percent	2 minutes
Work interval 3 (3.5 mph)	8 percent	1 minute
Rest interval 3 (3.5 mph)	0 percent	1 minute
Work interval 4 (3.5 mph)	6 percent	2 minutes
Rest interval 4 (3.5 mph)	0 percent	2 minutes
Work interval 5 (3.5 mph)	4 percent	2 minutes
Rest interval 5 (3.5 mph)	0 percent	2 minutes

(continued)

Table 16-2 *(continued)*		
Workout Segment	*Incline*	*Time*
Work interval 6 (3.5 mph)	4 percent	2 minutes
Cool-down (3.0 mph)	0 percent	5 minutes
Total time		30 minutes

Posture walk

What it is: A posture walk is any pace at which you concentrate on your walking form and technique.

The treadmill advantage: Although you need to pay attention to your form whenever you're walking, posture walks, as I call them, are a time to really home in on each aspect of your walking form. On a posture walk, you go through a head-to-toe checklist in your head and make adjustments accordingly. This process helps you know what good walking form feels like so that you eventually perform many of these good habits unconsciously.

Posture walks are probably more effective on a treadmill than they are anywhere else because you don't have to worry about avoiding passing cars, sidestepping curious dogs, or stepping off a curb.

How to do it: After a warm-up, move into your workout pace and start mentally going through the following form checklist. After you reach the bottom of the checklist, start at the top and run through it again.

The perfect posture walk lasts for about 25 minutes, including a 5-minute warm-up and a 5-minute cool-down. If you're really taking it seriously and concentrating fully, each run through the list will take you 3 to 5 minutes, so a 25-minute workout allows for three to four run-throughs. You can also incorporate a posture walk within any other type of workout. You can also run through the checklist just once at any point in any workout if you want a quick refresher on form. I train my clients to go through their checklists at least once during every treadmill workout they do.

- ✔ **Head and neck:** Your head should be perfectly centered between your shoulders, and your neck should feel relaxed. Focus on relaxing all the tension you hold in your head and neck; that means relaxing your jaw, mouth, and forehead. Imagine that your head is very light and easy to hold upright.

- ✔ **Shoulders and chest:** Your shoulders should be down and relaxed, and your chest and rib cage should be gently lifted and "square." Imagine that you have a puppet string attached to the center of your chest and the puppeteer is pulling lightly upward.

✔ **Arms and hands:** Bend your elbows to 90 degrees. Cup your hands as if you are holding a potato chip that you don't want to crush. Be sure to drive your elbows straight back so that they skim your waist as your arms move.

✔ **Abs and lower back:** Pull your abs in but don't force it. Strive for a natural but relaxed curve in your lower back.

✔ **Hips and thighs:** Power your leg movements from your hips rather than from your thighs alone. Bend your forward knee slightly upon impact.

✔ **Ankles and feet:** Relax your ankles. Strike heel first and roll through: heel-ball-toe. Think about pushing the treadmill away from you with your feet.

✔ **Breathing and heart rate:** Take deep, regular breaths and think about controlling the beat of your heart to match your steady breathing.

How to use the panel: Note changes and difficulties in your walking form at various speeds and inclines. If you have trouble with your form when you're walking faster or uphill, do most of your posture walk at this level. This technique can help make you a better walker whether you walk indoors or out.

Tuning out

When all is said and done, you may find it boring to monitor your treadmill panel on a regular basis. Although doing one or two "tune in" workouts a week is important, I'm all for using the treadmill as a great escape. Where else can you walk without having to worry about the environment around you? To this end, I suggest some "zone out" strategies in the following sections.

Watch TV

In many of my gyms, 3 p.m. is a popular workout time because a large group (not all women by the way!) comes in to see what's happening on *General Hospital*. In one of our other gyms, we have a VCR hooked up to every TV in front of each treadmill, and clients rent movies to watch while they work out. If they don't have time to watch the entire movie at once, the trainers keep track of where they are so that clients can watch the movie in installments.

Most people watch at least an hour or two of TV a week. Why not work your schedule around your favorite TV show? It helps the time pass and keeps you up-to-date with your favorite small-screen characters — whether you follow the nightly news or Mulder and Scully on *The X-Files*.

Listen to music

Whether it's the Starland Vocal Band or Puff Daddy, listen to whatever gets your adrenaline pumping and helps you keep up a good pace.

If you work out in a gym or health club, it may pipe in music. That's great if you happen to like the selections, but chances are, you may not. I recommend bringing your own headphones or portable CD player and playing music that you find motivating.

For safety reasons, a treadmill is the only place I recommend using headphones. When you walk outdoors, listening to your personal stereo prevents you from being aware of your surroundings and any potential dangers.

Several of my clients make custom tapes of their favorite songs and then share them with other clients. They try to use a mix of fast and slow songs to match each part of their workouts. When my mom walks, she listens to books on tape.

Talk to a friend

Take side-by-side treadmills next to a friend and dish the latest dirt to make time fly by. Just make sure that you're both working out hard enough so that your conversation is a little breathless. If your walking intensity is too high to carry on a conversation, you're probably working out too hard.

The strategy of talking to a treadmill neighbor backfired on my friend Hope. She once had the misfortune of working out next to someone who had just graduated from college with a psychology degree. After 25 minutes of unsolicited psychoanalysis, Hope cut her treadmill workout short and excused herself.

I often keep my headphones handy in case I'm not feeling particularly sociable. If I see someone I don't feel like talking to making a beeline for a neighboring treadmill, I quickly stick the headphones in my ears. Even if I don't listen to anything, I pretend that I'm totally occupied.

Surf the Web

I thought I had seen everything until I recently saw some new products that feature a computer screen rather than the regular treadmill control panel. Two products, Net Pulse and Internet Fitness Environment (IFE), provide a variety of distractions, including access to the Internet, e-mail, TV, CDs, radio, and video games. You can write a memo while you walk up a hill, catch the latest movie on pay per view, or chat with your Internet knitting group. (Your workout stats are displayed in a small box at the bottom of the screen.)

Personally, I don't want to check my e-mail while I'm working out. But I do love having 500 TV channels and all the latest music releases at my disposal. Right now, Internet integration with fitness equipment is available only at high-end gyms. But I think such features will become more common as technology becomes less expensive and more people accept computers as an integral part of their lives.

Six Steps to Treadmill Safety

Treadmills are among the easiest aerobic machines to use. Still, you do need to know a few things about safe treadmill use.

- ✔ **Use those safety features.** If your treadmill has an automatic stop, the option to code out nonauthorized users, or some other safety feature, take advantage of it.

- ✔ **Place your treadmill in a safe place.** If you have children, put your treadmill in a separate room that you can lock so they don't think it's a toy to play with. When the treadmill is in use, watch for children, pets, or clumsy spouses walking into the moving belt. (My dog walked into a moving treadmill belt once. Only once.) When you're not on the tread-mill, make sure that the belt is stopped. Don't leaving it running unat-tended — even for bathroom or phone breaks.

- ✔ **Straddle the belt when you start out.** Always place one foot on either side of the belt as you turn on the machine. Then step on the belt only after you determine that it's moving at the slow set-up speed. Most treadmills have safety features that prevent them from starting out at breakneck speeds, but don't take any chances.

- ✔ **Use the handrails sparingly.** Holding on for balance is okay when you're finding out how to use the machine, but let go as soon as you feel comfortable. You move more naturally if you swing your arms freely. If you must hold on to the front rails to charge up a hill or maintain a speed, you have the treadmill set at too high an intensity. Over-reliance on the handrails can overstrain your elbows and shoulders and reduces the amount of calories you burn during a workout.

- ✔ **Keep your eyes forward.** Your feet tend to follow your eyes, so if you focus on what's in front of you, you usually walk straight ahead instead of veering off to the side. Also, try to stay in the center of the belt rather than all the way toward the back or front. If you stay too close to the front, your foot can catch on the motor cover and trip you up; if you walk too close to the back, you may slide right off.

- ✔ **Expect to feel disoriented.** The first few times you use a treadmill, you may feel dizzy when you get off. Your body is just wondering why the ground suddenly stopped moving. Most people experience this vertigo only once or twice, but be prepared to hold on to something for a few moments when you hop off so that you don't fall over.

Treadmill classes

Picture this: Forty people are walking and running on treadmills while an instructor barks out instructions and encouragement. The guided jaunts involve climbing up inclines and sprinting toward imaginary finish lines. World-class runners sweat beside beginning walkers. And even though they are all doing the same general program, each person is working at his or her own personal workout intensity.

I have to give the credit for the concept of treadmill classes to my friend Ellen Abbott, the Boston Athletic Club's walking and running director. She created treading classes about four years ago in response to members' comments about the tedium of working out on the treadmill. These classes were an instant hit because they took the most popular piece of exercise equipment in the gym and gave it some pizzazz.

When Ellen presented treading at a recent World International Dance Exercise Association (IDEA) conference in California, it caused a sensation among exercise instructors. If your local gym doesn't already have a similar program, it probably will soon. Star Trac Treadmill has also rolled out its group class treadmill program, known as Trekking. My company, Plus One, calls its program MillWork.

Chapter 17

All Roads Lead to Fitness

*N*ot all walking routes follow the straight and narrow. Your walking program may take you to the far ends of the earth or to the nearest shopping mall. That's the beauty and flexibility of walking for exercise.

In this chapter, you get the scoop on all types of non-garden-variety walking scenarios, terrain, and circumstances that you're likely to encounter at some point during your walking career. You find out how to cope with the ever-changing landscape beneath your feet. You also figure out when you need to modify your technique, use specialized equipment, or take specific steps to avoid injury.

Hill, Yes!

Does the thought of climbing up a hill during your workout make you want to walk the other way? Perhaps you're suffering from *hillophobia,* my term for a common disorder that makes you quake with fear every time your feet meet with an incline. If you have such a problem, relax. The secret to walking hills is not to let them get the upper hand.

Instead of treating a hill as a sworn enemy, look at it as an opportunity to improve your fitness level and increase your walking prowess. Here are a few hill facts to give you extra incentive to take each climb in stride:

- For every additional 5 percent of incline (a modest rise in the landscape), you burn an extra 3 to 5 calories per minute, depending on your speed and effort level. That may not sound like a lot, but put it in perspective. The average person burns about 200 calories walking on a flat surface. If about half that distance consists of hills, the total calorie burn jumps to an average of 275 calories.

- Walking hills is a good way to increase the intensity of your workout without walking faster.

- Climbing hills strengthens the front of your thighs (the quadriceps and hip flexors), which may not get worked as hard when you walk on flat surfaces. And, because you must take smaller, lighter steps, hill work is a good alternative to sprints and fast walking to build overall leg strength. Increased leg strength also means greater endurance because you'll experience less leg fatigue.

- Because you have to lift your leg higher to walk up a hill, your buttocks muscles get more involved. That extra lift helps to tone and shape your entire lower body, especially your buttocks.

Going up

Uphill walking form is somewhat different from the walking form you use on flat surfaces. Follow these tips when walking uphill:

- Lean slightly forward.

- Let your hips and buttocks assist your thighs as much as possible.

- Use an arm swing that's relaxed and perhaps a little more forceful than usual, but not over-exaggerated. Your arm movement should mimic the arm movements used to pole in cross-country skiing.

- Instead of taking longer strides to keep you moving onward and upward, take quicker, shorter ones, lifting your knee no higher than 6 inches. The idea is to bustle, not bound, upward.

As you climb, aim to keep your intensity level on par with the rest of your workout. To gauge this, you can either strap on a heart rate monitor, do an occasional pulse check, or do this simple talk test: If you can carry on a breathless conversation, you're walking at the right pace.

 You can also monitor your breathing rhythm to judge intensity during uphill walking. Take two steps per inhale and two steps per exhale. If you find yourself breathing faster than this 2:2 pattern, it's a clear signal that you need to slow down. If your breath-to-footfall ratio is slower than 2:2, you're probably not working hard enough and should pick up the pace.

Aerobic imagery

Looking at a hill as one huge, insurmountable task may be self-defeating. Because hills often become larger and more intimidating in your mind's eye than they actually are, you may find it easier to make your peace with a hill by dividing it up and attacking it one section at a time.

Try focusing on a tree or some other sturdy object that's partway up the hill. Visualize yourself throwing an imaginary rope around the object and using it to "pull" yourself upward. Each time you reach your landmark, cast another imaginary rope up the hill. Before you know it, you'll reach the summit — marveling at how easy it was to get there after all.

Going down

Surprisingly, you're most likely to be injured when walking down a hill. Because you hit the ground harder as you move down a hill, stress and impact on your joints and muscles are multiplied. You're also thrown a little farther forward than normal, making it difficult to call upon large amounts of muscle to support your body weight. Knee injuries and quadriceps strains are the most common pitfalls of poor downhill form.

To lessen your chance of injury, follow these tips when walking downhill:

- ✔ Walk in a relaxed glide instead of careening out of control until you reach the bottom. Take small, fast steps, letting each footstrike flow smoothly into the next.

- ✔ Don't try to fight gravity by leaning back and putting on the brakes. Lean forward slightly so that your torso stays perpendicular to the road surface.

- ✔ If the downhill is very steep, use a technique called *switchbacking*, in which you snake from side to side across a hill.

  It's best to steer clear of extreme downward slopes whenever possible. The steepest downhill you train on shouldn't be as inclined as the steepest hill you're able to go up.

Creating your own hills

What if you're ready to hit the high roads but you live in an area that's flatter than a pancake? Do your climbing on a treadmill. Many treadmills incline up to a 25 percent grade, and some actually decline to simulate downhills. (Turn to Chapter 16 to find out more about treadmills.)

If you don't have access to a treadmill, you'll have to get even more imaginative about creating mountains out of no hills. Is there a bridge near you that arches upward to the center? How about the rolling hills of a golf course? I have one client who lives in Kansas, one of the flatter places on earth. Early every Sunday morning, when there's very little car activity, she uses the up ramps of her parking garage to do her hill training.

Strolling on the Beach

The beach is a terrific place to laze around on an oversized towel and soak up some rays, but it's also a wonderful place to walk. Besides offering beautiful scenery, the beach is a place where you can walk for miles without obstacles. However, walking on the beach is not without pitfalls.

You may think that dry sand is easy on your joints because it is soft and giving. It is not. When you step down on sand, your feet sink below a level surface, and your joints, especially your ankles and knees, have to work extra hard to lift your foot up and out for the next step. Walking in dry sand is more challenging aerobically as well. You've probably noticed that you may feel a little out of breath just from walking around looking for a place to put down your towel. Definitely try to avoid walking on dry sand for extended periods of time if you aren't very fit or have any chronic ankle, knee, or lower back problems.

Do your beach walking along the edge of the shoreline where the sand is firm and wet. Your feet will still sink down to some extent — not enough to stress out your joints, but just enough to make your workout more strenuous. I like to walk barefoot close enough to the water's edge for the waves to wash over my feet. I find the saltwater especially healing if I have blisters or cuts on my feet.

But depending on the beach, going barefoot isn't always the smartest option. Pieces of broken shells, glass, and other sharp debris can cut and damage your feet. If this is the case, keep your walking shoes on and walk a little farther away from the edge of the water. Try to avoid getting your shoes soaked. Wet, soggy shoes are uncomfortable and can promote blisters and a whole host of other foot problems.

Here is some other advice to consider before you hit the sand:

✔ **Sand reflects sunlight and absorbs heat, so wearing sunscreen for your beach walks is especially important.** Reapply sunscreen frequently, especially if you've been sweating or you've just come out of the water. Don't forget these easy-to-overlook spots that come to your attention only after they are burned to a crisp: your ears, in between your toes, along the edges of your bathing suit, and the back of your knees and neck.

✔ **Don't forget the bug spray.** When a grape-sized horsefly takes a bite out of you, it's like getting pinched by a really aggressive aunt. Ouch! Look for a product that is a combined bug repellent and sunscreen.

✔ **Wear a hat and sunglasses to protect your face from UV rays.** Such protective gear lessens the possibility of wrinkling and premature aging of your skin and also helps reduce your risk of skin cancer.

✔ **Avoid walking during the hottest part of the day, between 11 a.m. and 2 p.m.** Plan your beach walk around the sunrise or sunset to avoid heat-related complications.

✔ **If you do a lot of beach walking, consider purchasing a pair of aqua shoes.** Several companies make a special shoe for walking on wet surfaces. Large shoe companies make an aqua sock or slipper that is made of a quick-dry nylon mesh; these also have extra-good traction to prevent slipping and sliding. My favorite aqua shoes are made by a company called Ryka. Besides being quick-dry and sturdy, they have little drains in the bottoms so that water and debris drain quickly. I once brought along a pair on a rafting and hiking trip to the Grand Canyon. They caused such a sensation with the other people on my trip that I gave them away to one of my fellow travelers.

✔ **Be sure to drink plenty of water.** In bright sunlight, you will dehydrate much more quickly than usual. And you'll dehydrate even more quickly if you walk seaside, thanks to the salty air. Bring along a water bottle and sip it frequently as you stroll. Keep it in your ice chest under a shady umbrella between walks.

✔ **If you are using your everyday walking shoes to walk on the beach, make sure that you dry them thoroughly and take great pains to remove every grain of sand from the inside of them.** Remove the insoles and brush them vigorously. One unfortunately placed grain of sand can cause skin irritation, blisters, and discomfort.

Walking in Circles

Many walkers prefer to do their thing on a track for the following reasons:

✔ It provides an exactly measured distance.

✔ The surface is usually cinder, rubber, or some other type of material that's springy and easy on your joints.

✔ Many tracks have nearby bathroom and locker room facilities.

✔ Most tracks have a water fountain that works all year-round.

Outdoor tracks usually measure 400 meters or 440 yards. Four trips around the track equal one mile or close to it. Because you know the exact distance, a track is an ideal place to do a time trial. To get an idea of what your standard walking pace is, use a stopwatch, or chronograph, to time how long it takes you to do four loops. If walking four laps takes you 20 minutes, you know that your pace is a 20-minute mile or, put another way, you walk at a speed of 3 miles per hour. This information gives you an indication about how far you walk when you don't have a measured course. Knowing your pace also gives you an indication of how many calories you burn during a workout. (See the tables in Chapters 7 through 10 to figure out your calorie usage.)

Unfortunately, many people find that walking in circles is as boring as it sounds. To offset the monotony, try walking with a friend. Listening to headphones is fine, too, as long as it is broad daylight and plenty of people are around.

For your own safety, avoid walking on a track when no one else is around or when it's dark. Stay aware of your surroundings, including the other people who are working out. Because most tracks are fenced in, if you get into trouble, you can feel like you're trapped in a cage.

Most tracks are slightly angled or banked, so your inside knee has more pressure placed on it, especially on the turns. Reverse your direction every mile so that you don't wind up with overuse injuries on the inside leg. However, reversing direction isn't always allowed, especially on tracks that aren't very wide or that are especially crowded. Usually you have to move in a clockwise direction on some days and counterclockwise direction on others. If the track you use follows this policy, try to plan your workouts so that you aren't always going in the same direction during every workout.

Indoor tracks are a nice alternative for indoor walkers who can't abide the idea of walking on a treadmill. Indoor tracks don't have a standard size, but most are considerably smaller than the standard outdoor track. They are extremely banked and have tight, narrow turns. For this reason, reversing directions as often as possible is even more important. An indoor track is not the best place to train if you have achy knees. In fact, as much as I hate to discourage anyone from taking full advantage of a safe, measured place to walk, I must advise against walking on an indoor track if you have chronic knee problems.

Track etiquette

If you walk on a track, study these rules and regulations. They'll keep you on friendly terms with other tracksters.

- A standard track usually has four lanes. Speedier movers use the inside lanes, meaning that runners generally occupy the two innermost lanes and walkers use the two outermost lanes.

- When walking with a friend, walking in lanes side by side is okay. However, if the track is crowded, walk single file to allow other exercisers to pass more easily.

- When passing someone, don't just sneak up behind her and blow by. When you are about an arm's length away, call out in a friendly tone, "On your left" or "On your right." This is a track insider's shorthand for "I'm passing you on the left (or right) side."

- Don't stash your belongings on the edge of the track or on bleacher steps, where they may be in the way of other exercisers. When lockers aren't available, I place my stuff on the grass in the center of the track. That way, I can keep an eye on everything at all times, just in case someone tries to make off with my things.

- Don't hog a lane to do your stretches or calisthenics. Warm up and cool down in the infield, the bleachers, or some other area where you won't interfere with other walkers and runners.

- Obey track hours as well as all other rules and regulations. For example, some tracks do not allow pets. Other tracks close for special events or at certain times of the day to allow school athletes private workout time.

Hitting the Trails

Hiking can take the boredom out of walking. It gets you out in the fresh air and allows you to commune with nature. Many of my clients plan weekend hikes as a reward for working hard all week. Hiking gives their weekday workouts a purpose and direction: They train hard so that they can go for longer, more challenging hikes on the weekend. Even if you live in an urban area, you're probably just a 1- or 2-hour drive from some scenic walks.

For the best local hikes in your area, check with your parks department, Chamber of Commerce, or local walking or hiking group. Sometimes neighborhood bookstores have accurate and detailed maps of local trails. At a large hiking and mountaineering shop in New York City, I found a terrific book that details the trails throughout upstate New York. I love this book because it gives me not only the mileage and the average hiking time for each trail but also the history of the area and the names of landmarks. With a little luck and detective work, you can probably find a similar book for trails in your area.

I am an avid hiker. I love to hear the birds singing, the sound of a running stream, and the soft crunch of pine needles beneath my feet. One of my fondest memories is the 10-day hiking trip my husband and I took along the coast of southern Wales. The Coastal Path we walked along is famous for its cliffs and ocean view on one side and its farms and ancient castles on the other. If you ever get the chance to take such a trip, I highly recommend it.

Playing it safe

Because most hikes take place off the beaten path, so to speak, make safety a high priority. Here are some tips to keep your hike safe and enjoyable:

- **Never attempt a trail that's beyond your ability.** Trails can range from pleasant, pine-needle-covered dirt paths to rocky, nearly vertical scrambles. Make sure that you know what you're getting into before it's too late. Remember that you can't exactly hail a cab if you become too exhausted to continue.

- **Plan your route.** Bring maps and directions. Have some indication of about how long a round-trip hike will take, including rest stops and lunch breaks. Start early enough to make it out of the woods by dusk. Always let someone know where you are going and when you expect to be back. If there is a trail book, be sure to sign in.

- **Check weather reports.** Take them seriously and prepare for the worst. You don't want to get caught unexpectedly in a thunderstorm or a sudden heavy snowfall. I recommend bringing extra rain and/or snow gear along just in case. Carrying the extra weight is a pain, but if you need it, you'll be grateful that you lugged it along. If the forecast calls for severe weather, consider skipping your hike and going another day. For winter hiking, consider snowshoeing or cross-country skiing as a hiking alternative.

- **Bring along a first aid kit that includes bandages, antiseptic, and a snake bite kit.** Many people scoff at this advice, especially if they plan to be out for only an hour or two, but believe me, my first aid kit has come in handy more than once. I bought a small one for around $10. When I use something from it, I replace it as soon as I get home so that I don't forget.

- **Bring a snack and plenty of water.** Drink frequently and fuel up to keep your energy steady for the trail ahead. Many hikers like to munch on granola or a mix of peanuts and raisins known as gorp (shorthand for Good Old Raisins and Peanuts). Any lowfat snack will do though, as long as it doesn't get smooshed and mashed up in your bag.

- **If you heed just one piece of advice I offer you about hiking in the woods, please make it this: Never hike alone.** It takes so little for something to go wrong. You may lose your way or fall and injure your-self. If you're alone, there is no telling when you will be found.

Even though I know better, I once broke my own Golden Rule of Hiking — never hike alone. I was spending a few days alone in our country house in upstate New York when I decided to take my greyhound, Zoomer, on a familiar trail that I have been hiking for years. Just as I reached the top of the mountain, I heard a noise behind me and turned to see a man walking up behind me with a loaded shotgun. My heart nearly leapt out of my chest, and I instantly began imagining the worst. Luckily, Zoomer is a large, very imposing dog; he began barking and snapping at the man, who put his hands in the air and backed off. It turns out that he was a friendly hunter taking in some target practice. But what if he wasn't? I was a 3-hour walk to the nearest house. What could I have done to protect myself? I can honestly say that I will never go hiking alone again, even with my trusty watchdog to protect me!

Knowing what equipment you'll need

Hiking requires highly specialized equipment that differs from the equipment you need for other types of fitness walking. Here's some advice to help you get started:

- ✔ **Hiking shoes:** Whereas fitness walking shoes are flexible in the forefoot to allow for maximum bendability in the front of the shoe, hiking shoes are more substantial in the forefoot and a bit stiffer overall. Hiking is done at a much slower pace than walking, so toe-off is minimal. The rigidity is required for traction, foot stability, and protection from rocks and other debris. Even if your hiking shoes are waterproof or water-resistant, it never hurts to treat them with a waterproofing product to ensure that your feet don't get soggy.

- ✔ **Hiking clothes:** Poison oak, poison ivy, and ticks carrying Lyme disease are a big worry in a large part of the country from March through November. That's why most experts recommend covering as much of your body as you can, even when it's hot. Be sure to tuck your pants legs into your walking shoes or boots and wear a hat. Wear a cap to prevent ticks from embedding themselves into your scalp, too.

    You probably won't wear the same clothes you wear hiking as you do during your everyday walks. Specialized shirts, pants, and socks are available that are made especially for hikers; they are usually a bit more rugged than everyday walking wear. You should always carry foul weather gear with you, too, even if there isn't a cloud in the sky. Sometimes weather moves in quickly, and you don't want to get caught in an unexpected downpour without rain gear.

- ✔ **Bug repellent:** Wear plenty of bug spray. Brands like Off and DEET repel both ticks and mosquitoes. Be careful with these products, though; some of my clients complain of skin rashes and other reactions from wearing this stuff. Test it out on a small area of skin and see whether you develop a reaction. When in doubt, read the label on the product you're using.

✔ **Hiking pack:** For 1- to 2-hour hikes, you can probably get by with a simple fanny pack that cinches around your waist. For longer hikes, wear a day-hiking backpack and stock it with a snack, extra socks, and a first aid kit. If you are hiking for more than a day, I recommend getting a larger, sturdy hiking pack with a frame.

A good day-hiking pack has padded shoulder straps and conforms to the shape of your back. All straps should be fully adjustable so that you can customize the fit. The best ones have a waist cinch that helps take pressure off the lower back and shoulders and distributes more of the weight of the pack on your hips. Some also have a special pocket to hold your water bottle. Although dozens of excellent backpacks are available, I have had very good luck with Eagle Creek and Eastpak brand packs. They have a wide variety of shapes and sizes to choose from, most priced at under $50.

✔ **Walking poles:** These are optional, but you may find them very beneficial. Walking poles help you power up hills and steady yourself on loose gravel and dirt, downhill slopes, and rocky trails. Good poles are adjustable in height, offer some sort of shock absorption, and have comfortable grips. For a detailed description of walking poles, see Chapter 18.

For more detailed information on hiking equipment, contact your local parks department or hiking group.

Mall Walking

I like to think of shopping malls as "tread malls." By clocking off miles in a mall, you get climate control, mall security, and a clean, safe surface on which to exercise. You can combine shopping and companionship with a dash of fitness. What fun!

For many people, doing laps around a mall is far more interesting than walking circles around a track or logging miles on a treadmill. The idea is a boon to older people who need a safe place to walk and for people in areas where walking outside is difficult. Many people who participate in my weekly online chat tell me that they prefer walking in a mall because they are just getting back into shape or they have limited mobility. For them, malls provide plenty of seating if they need to take a break. If they get into trouble, they can always call for security or get help from a fellow mall walker or shopper. Plus, window-shopping while walking makes the time go by faster.

Many formal mall walking groups meet before the mall opens or after it closes. But you can mall walk at any time of the day if the urge hits you. You don't have to confine yourself to a mall, either. When my mother gets bored, she walks the aisles of the supermarket because she finds it more relaxing to go food shopping than window-shopping. I have a client who likes to walk through the large 24-hour superstores because, she says, "there's something different around every corner, so I never get bored."

Joining a mall walking club is simple. Usually all you have to do is go to the main information desk and fill out an application. At no cost or for a nominal fee, the club provides you with little incentives like maps, mileage charts, schedules, and special discount cards. Some larger mall clubs offer walkers' "credit cards" that, when run through reader machines, log mileage and award prizes.

Check with your local mall to see whether it has a formal walking club. If it doesn't, why not start one of your own? Often, a mall will advertise it for you for free on one of its bulletin boards or its Web site. You can also contact the National Organization of Mall Walkers for information and details about clubs in your area and the steps you need to take to charter your own. This organization also sends free information packets to members. For more information, see the list of resources in the appendix.

Water Walking

At times, submerging your walking program in water that's above your waist or even deeper makes a lot of sense. Water walking is the perfect break from the pounding of everyday training on terra firma. It's a wonderful way to keep active if you're nursing an injury. And when the outdoor temperature climbs into the 90s, it's a refreshing version of earthbound walking. Water walking is also an excellent aerobic and calorie burning workout; you can burn up to 550 calories an hour walking in the water.

Water walking can also help correct muscle imbalances. Walking on land emphasizes the muscles in the front and back of your thighs. Walking in water works your upper body equally as hard as your lower body because water gives all your submerged muscles 12 to 14 times the resistance of air.

Taking a water walking or running class is a good way to get a handle on form and technique. Many colleges, universities, and high schools offer relatively inexpensive classes to the public. YMCAs, Jewish Community Centers, and public pools may also offer these types of classes.

There are two types of water walking: deep water and shallow water. Here's a description of each type:

   ✔ **Deep water walking** is done in a pool or any other calm body of water where your feet don't touch the bottom. During deep water walking, you mimic land-based walking movements such as walking up hills, walking sprints, and backwards walking.

Although it is not absolutely necessary, I recommend that you wear a flotation vest or belt. This device keeps you afloat and holds you in a relatively stable condition in the water so that you can concentrate on your form instead of on keeping yourself afloat. If your pool doesn't have a buoy vest and you want to give water walking a try before you invest the $50 or so on a flotation device of your own, you can try propping a Styrofoam weight under each arm to keep yourself afloat. Most pools have them. Stick them firmly under your arms so that they don't interfere with your arm swing and so they keep you relatively stationary in the water.

I like the Wet Vest and the Wet Belt flotation devices made by Bioenergetics. Both are adjustable for a customized fit. They also minimize the water buffalo look that some flotation devices give you, thanks to their streamlined designs.

✔ **Shallow water walking** is done in thigh- to chest-high water where your feet still can touch the bottom. If your space is limited, you can tether yourself to the side of the pool with a stretchy band or a bungee cord so that you can keep moving your body without actually having to move through the pool. Otherwise, walk the pool back and forth widthwise, driving your arms and legs as hard as you can. Don't worry about speed. You won't move very fast. But you will work up a sweat and tire out quickly. I recommend starting with a few short intervals with a minute or two of rest in between and gradually increasing from there.

To prevent chafed feet, wear special aqua shoes or an old pair of sneakers to walk in shallow water. I have a pair of Ryka Aqua Sport shoes that are designed for just this purpose. They have little "drains" in the bottoms and sides so that they never feel bloated or heavy with water. They also dry within 15 minutes. Nike, Reebok, and most other major shoe manufacturers also make aqua shoes.

Watered-down heart rate

If you take your pulse during any type of water walking session, you'll probably find that it doesn't get as high as it does during land-based training that feels similar in difficulty. That's because your maximum heart rate in the water is generally 8 percent to 10 percent lower than your normal maximum heart rate.

Scientists speculate people have a lower heart rate in the water because the pressure of water on the legs helps "push" blood back up toward your heart, flooding it between beats and increasing the amount of blood ejected by the heart with each beat. Tremendously high heart rates aren't needed to get the blood pumping into the working muscles. If you typically keep track of your heart rate during your walks, it may not provide an accurate picture during water walking. You probably can get a more accurate picture of exercise intensity simply by aiming for an effort level that roughly feels the same as the walking you do on land.

Part IV
The Part of Tens

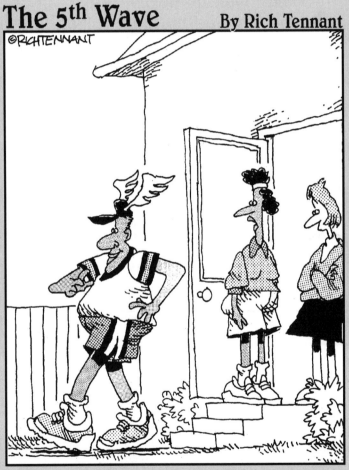

The 5th Wave   By Rich Tennant

©RICHTENNANT

"He's lost 12 lbs. and 3 inches from his waist. Now, if I can just get him to lose that hat."

In this part . . .

1 carry on the *For Dummies* tradition of grouping key information into fun, easy-to-skim lists of ten. In Chapter 18, you find out about ten great gadgets to check out. Some of these gadgets help you burn more calories and prevent falls, while other products help keep you safe. The next chapter gives you the lowdown on ten great walking resources, including which magazines are a must-read for walkers and which catalogs have the best walking clothes. Chapter 20 focuses on ten surefire ways to keep your walking program motivating and interesting — including surfing the Net while you walk or taking a stroll with your best canine buddy.

Chapter 18

Ten Great Gadgets for Walkers

*O*ne of the beauties of using walking as a form of exercise is that it is wonderfully uncomplicated and lacking in any major necessary accoutrements, save a good pair of walking shoes. Still, if you're a gadget freak like me, you may find it hard to resist trying out at least a few accessories in the name of bettering your efforts.

In this chapter, I suggest ten gadgets that you may find useful in your walking program. Many of them add some upper body resistance, thereby increasing muscle usage and calorie burn. Others give you information about your walking program. Still others help make walking easier or more enjoyable. You're bound to find one of them irresistible. I own them all!

Taking a Pole

When I was hiking in upstate New York about ten years ago, I noticed ski hikers using ski poles to power themselves up the trail. I later found out that serious mountaineers and hikers have been using ski poles for decades as a means of balance and support, especially while navigating steep or uneven terrain. Just recently, I've noticed fitness walkers using poles, too.

The more I find out about ski poles, the more I like the idea of using them as a walking tool. Because poles don't force your arm and shoulder muscles to check the momentum of your arm swing, they're safer than hand weights. By planting the poles vigorously and pushing back with them each time you stride, you use the poles to create resistance against the ground. This movement brings your arms, shoulders, chest, and back muscles into play. All these muscles work in a steady, controlled manner, resulting in less stress to the connective tissues of the shoulder.

Poles aren't too shabby in the calorie burn department either: Studies show that when you walk with poles, you can burn up to 33 percent more calories even at slower paces. By the way, this is not the case with hand weights: Surprisingly, some studies have shown that you actually burn fewer calories when you walk with hand weights because the slower pace you need to walk to keep them under control offsets the increased calorie burn you get from using them.

And, if those ski hikers I saw are any example, I think that the poles propel you forward a little faster, especially when climbing hills. They help guide you going downhill as well.

I don't recommend using poles everywhere, all the time. They work best for walks on natural terrain such as dirt and trails. Though I have seen some people using them on asphalt and cement, I find that using poles on such surfaces is a little jarring. Poles are fine for cinder tracks, but don't use poles on rubberized tracks because they poke holes in the surface.

The best walking poles I've tried are the Exerstriders, which sell for about $60. They look like ski poles but have special rubber tips for shock absorption and to aid in arm push-off. Comfortable handgrips and wrist straps allow you to keep your hands relaxed. The poles also telescope to the proper height. I especially like the instruction booklet and video that come with them; both offer tons of technique tips to help you use the poles most efficiently. The video stars Tom Rutlin, the inventor of Exerstriding, whose enthusiasm for his product really comes across.

Wiping Out Calories

This is definitely one of my weirder suggestions and one you won't see on the Home Shopping Network any time soon: Wave two small hand towels as you walk. I know this advice sounds odd, but a recent University of Houston study suggests that dangling a small towel from each hand and, using your normal arm swing, flapping them in the air as you walk can burn up to 70 extra calories an hour. The reason? As you wave the towels back and forth, they create a small wind current so that you have to work harder to swing your arms.

I admit, you may feel kind of silly walking around the neighborhood whipping towels through the air. After reading the study, I experimented with this technique at night on a back road with no one around. I can tell you — goofiness aside — that it really works.

I don't recommend any specific brand, weight, or color of towel. I used old blue wash cloths, which worked just fine.

If you can tolerate the stares and comments, you may want to try using towels first, before you purchase any of the other resistance-adding gadgets I recommend in this chapter. If nothing else, they're free.

Measuring Your Heart Rate

Your heart rate provides the most useful tool for determining whether you are over- or under-doing it. Unfortunately, the traditional method of placing a finger on your neck or wrist to count the number of times your heart beats in a minute isn't very convenient or precise.

"I have trouble finding my pulse or counting the beats without losing track," my cousin Margie always complains. And taking her heart rate while on the move? Forget about it! "I can't do it without stumbling over my feet," Margie says. Clumsy cousins aside, stopping your walk for a pulse check breaks your rhythm, so your heart rate immediately slows and accuracy goes out the window.

Enter the heart rate monitor. Once a heart rate monitor was a bulky device requiring half a dozen wires and electrodes, but today's models are light-weight, wireless, and extremely user-friendly. Many new models also sport some innovative, high-tech features. For instance, some monitors now speak to you, telling you what your heart rate is and even giving advice on whether to pick up the pace or not. One model, made by Polar, beeps to remind you to wear it if you haven't used it in the past few days.

All walkers should consider using a heart rate monitor at least some of the time.

Without regular monitoring, you may think that you're exercising at a certain intensity, but in fact, you may not be. You may discover that you're not working hard enough, or, if you're trying to take it easy, the monitor may indicate a need to slow down. This instantaneous precision allows you to fine-tune workout levels. (See Chapter 5 for more details on target heart rate zones.)

If you thrive on feedback, tracking the rhythms of your heart can be motivational as well. As you get fitter, your heart doesn't have to work as hard at a given workload, so monitoring your pulse lets you know whether you're getting in better shape. Monitoring also tells you how fast your heart rate recovers at the end of your workout and between hard-driving intervals. The more quickly your heart rate drops, the better condition your heart is in.

Cousin Margie was amazed when her heart rate plummeted after doing the same treadmill program over a period of weeks. When she first started, her heart rate monitor consistently signaled that her heart rate averaged in the high 160s during her 30-minute walk. But after a few weeks of doing the same program faithfully at least three days a week, she was averaging in the mid

140s. At that point, we knew it was time to design a walking program that was a little more challenging for her. Of course, heart rate was just another way of confirming that the program was indeed getting easier for her. The fact that her breathing was less labored, her legs felt springier, and she didn't feel as winded afterwards also were signs that she was ready for more.

Typical heart monitors measure your pulse in one of two ways. Photo-optic models clip onto your earlobe or fingertip and shine a beam of infrared light through your skin to measure the amount of blood pumped into your blood vessels; they relay this information to a digital screen or special wristwatch. This is an inexpensive, simple system, but not without its problems. Any relative motion between the sensor and finger causes highly erratic or false readings. Daylight, poor circulation, and high-intensity exercise may also skew precision.

I recommend buying the other type of heart rate monitor — an electro-cardio sensor — which operates on the same principle as a medical electrocardiogram (ECG). Using radio signals, it directly measures the electrical activity of the heart with a fairly high degree of accuracy. (Many electro-cardio sensors claim to be precise within one beat of a medical ECG.) A chest strap acts as a sort of electrode and transmits the information to a wristwatch receiver. Some styles also offer extra features such as a clock, timer, and a settable alarm that trips every time you wander out of your training range.

Polar is widely considered the best manufacturer of heart rate monitors. The most basic model, The Polar Beat strap-and-watch combo, costs about $50. It's perfect for an entry-level walker experimenting with pulse monitoring because the only thing it does is gauge heart rate. If you're looking to spend around 300 smackers for something that downloads information onto your PC, records lap times, and does everything but wash the dishes, the Polar Accurex Plus is the model for you. (The good news is that monitor prices are now lower because the market is so much more competitive.)

Treadmill users can now more easily use a heart rate monitor because most popular treadmills (like Trotter, Quinton, and Star Trac) now include a feature that reads your heart rate directly on the display panel. Though you don't have to wear the watch, you still have to wear the chest strap. But you don't have to raise your wrist up to your eyeball.

Polar also makes a special Heart Bra that allows you to thread the chest strap through the bottom band of the bra. My friend Mindy Solkin designed this Lycra sports bra, and when she first brought me one, I thought "So what." After one workout, I realized that the bra prevented the irritation I used to get from wearing the monitor underneath my bra, plus it held it in place for more accurate readings. Now, I always wear my Heart Bra whenever I wear my monitor. It costs about $30, which is right in line price-wise with other high-quality sports bras. You can find them in any good sports clothing store or order them from Polar's Web site.

Walking a Mile with a Camel

As much of a gadget freak as I am, I can't stand carrying anything in my hands when I walk or run. It makes me feel uncomfortable and unbalanced. For this reason, water bottles don't work for me. I'm not the only fussy drinker either — many other walkers and runners have told me that they feel the same way.

Because you must drink as often as possible when you walk, especially when it's hot, you have to find a comfortable way to carry water with you. If holding one or two water bottles in your hands or in a waist holster works for you, that's great. But if you can't stand all that sloshing and dripping, take a tip borrowed from our cycling and triathlon friends.

For years, cyclists have worn water reservoir devices that cinch around their waists or strap onto their backs in order to keep their hands free. Here's how these liquid pouches work: You fill up the reservoir with water and then thread the long, plastic, soft straw through your clothing so that the end is near your mouth. Instead of messing with a water bottle every time you need a drink, you simply turn and sip. It couldn't be easier or more convenient.

I'm now starting to see walkers and runners wear these same devices. I often wear one myself for long hikes, walks, and runs. I think liquid pouches help you stay better hydrated for two reasons. First of all, because they make water so accessible, you're likely to drink more. And because most of these reservoirs hold 20 to 90 ounces of liquid, you have more to drink. By comparison, standard water bottles hold anywhere from 8 to 16 ounces of liquid.

As much as I love wearing my liquid pouch, it takes some getting used to. You may need to use it on two to three walks before you're able to hook it up effortlessly and are comfortable with the feel and weight of it. But trust me, it's worth it. After you wear one a while, you'll love it.

Besides storing water, many liquid pouch models let you stuff your personal stereo, pager, pencil case, and all your other stuff in its storage pouches. I have one client who liked his so much he even wore it under his suit to work for a while!

Camelbak, Blackburn, Liquipac, and Traveling Light all make excellent water-fanny pack combos. Prices range from $30 to $100 depending on the size and number of pouches. Try a few on first and find the configuration that works best for you. Most good sporting good and camping stores sell them. You may save a little money by purchasing online or by catalog, but make sure that you know which model you're looking for.

Taking Time to Walk

One of the greatest advances in modern athletics is the $20 sports watch. Owning one is like having your own coach, cheerleader, and statistician on your wrist.

Today's sports watches go beyond simply telling you what time it is; they have a mind-boggling array of functions. Here's a list and description of just a few features that walkers find the most useful:

- **Stopwatch:** Even the most basic sports watches have a timer, stopwatch, or chronograph that measures your walk to the nearest hundredth of a second. Many walkers find it motivating to time the same route and keep track of improvements and "personal bests" or "personal records," the fastest time they have ever walked the same distance. (If you want to seem cool, refer to your personal record as simply your "PR." It makes you sound like a pro-in-the-know to your walking group and your kids.)

- **Lap timer:** The lap timer function is a useful tool for those who walk on tracks, do loops of the same distance, or race. By pressing the lap timer button on your watch, you freeze the time it takes you to walk one lap, but the timer still keeps going to track your overall time.

A one-lap time measurement is referred to as your *split time* or *split*. Splits give you a way of comparing one lap to another so that you know whether you're slowing down or speeding up.

Most sports watches store up to eight splits. Some of the fancier ones, like some models of the Timex Ironman, record up to 100.

- **A light:** You never realize how useful a light is until you don't have one. If you walk outdoors at night or early in the morning, you probably want to see how long you've been moving. Look for a watch that has a light that works while the chronograph runs so that you can view your elapsed time.

Here again, Timex, with its patented Indiglo light feature, has the edge over most other sports watches I've seen.

- **A comfortable watchband:** A flexible plastic watchband has it over a metal watchband because it allows you to sweat freely and doesn't pinch the skin. Thank goodness these bands now come in an array of colors, styles, and widths so that you don't have to settle for the wide ugly gray bands that were one of the few options up until a few years ago.

Swatch carries some really outstanding sports watches that are pretty enough to wear all the time.

- **All the rest:** If you want to spend between $70 to $200, you can own a watch that downloads all your information onto your computer, stores telephone numbers, and beeps in time with your walking cadence. Most walkers can probably live without all these fancy extras, but they are fun to have.

My father has a watch with all the optional extras; he tells everyone that he has a "Rolodex" watch. This impresses people who aren't listening very carefully because they think he's claiming to own a "Rolex" — one of the world's most expensive line of watches.

Lighting up Your Life

I am amazed at how many "stealth" walkers and runners I see out exercising in the dark. This is my term for people who dress in dark colors from head to toe and, intentionally or not, blend into the darkness. Besides running the real risk of getting hit by a car or cyclist, stealth walkers scare the life out of you because you are mere inches away from them before you realize that they're there.

For those who walk when it's dark, whether alone or in a pack, wearing reflectors or blinking lights is a must. Bright fluorescent or white clothing improves visibility at night.

Numerous clothing manufacturers make jackets, shirts, and tights with reflective panels or stripes. Most walking shoes also have some sort of reflective material on the sides, heels, or outers.

Sporting goods, cycling, and running shops sell reflective jackets, shirts, and lightweight vests that slip over your walking outfit. These increase your safety because they define your entire shape in the dark so that motorists recognize a person in their headlights. I also highly recommend placing cloth or plastic reflective tape and stickers directly on your jacket, shoes, hats, and gloves. This reflective material is cheap, weighs virtually nothing, is available in red or white for forward and rear use, and can be placed anywhere.

Jogalite makes a virtually unlimited array of reflective products — everything from cut-n-peel glow-in-the-dark tape to blinking lights that attach to your bag or clothing. Most of these reflectors and lights cost only a few dollars, wash well, and last for months. You can find Jogalite and other reflective products in sporting good and hardware stores. (Hint: They're usually considerably less expensive in stores like Home Depot or Wal-Mart.) You can also order them online.

Refreshing Your Sole

My friend Donna tells a story about lacing up a brand new pair of shoes, heading out the door, and promptly stepping into a deep, muddy puddle with her right foot only. "For weeks I walked with one clean shoe and one filthy one," she said, "I finally replaced them because they looked so stupid."

When you consider that a decent pair of walking shoes costs a minimum of $45 (and upwards of $120), you quickly realize that taking care of your shoes goes beyond vanity — it can extend their life span and save you money.

Though walking shoes can be worn for 500 to 1,000 miles before the cushioning in the midsole completely breaks down, most people toss them much sooner because of dirty uppers, sweat-eaten inners, or uneven wearing of the soles. That's where sole patching products and store-bought inserts come in handy. I use them as part of this three-step remedy to turn grungy footwear (both leather and cloth) into sparkling clean, like-new beauties:

1. **Machine wash up to four pairs of walking or athletic shoes in a full load using the short cycle and cold to warm water.**

   Remove and wash the insoles. (You may replace these in Step 3 depending on how worn they are.) Use a quarter cup of chlorine bleach or half cup of all-fabric bleach. Dry the shoes in a warm, shaded place.

   Machine washing restores a nearly new appearance and should kill the bacteria that thrives on sweat, but if you overwash, the midsoles will harden up. For this reason, you can get away with only one machine washing in the lifetime of each pair of shoes.

2. **Use a coarse-grade sandpaper to rough up the worn areas of the soles, especially at the heel and outer edges.**

3. **Apply two layers of a shoe patching product over the entire sole of shoe. I recommend Shoe Goo or Shoe Patch for this purpose. Both are available at large discount stores like Kmart or Wal-Mart for around $4 a tube.**

   These gluelike products form a clear, protective layer between the bottom of the shoe and the ground so that the soles don't wear as quickly. Apply thin, even layers and let each layer dry thoroughly before applying the next — otherwise you wind up with bumpy, uneven soles. Allow 2 hours of drying time between layers and 12 or more hours for final drying.

   Each shoe patch application lasts about 20 miles, depending on how heavy your footstrike is and how much you weigh. You can apply again and again for as long as you wear the shoes.

4. **Replace the shoe's insole with a $10 to $20 store-bought insert to enhance its shock absorption.**

   When adding a new insole, you may have to carefully trim them to the correct size and shape with a pair of nail scissors to prevent crowding your toes.

You can buy inserts in drugstores, running shops, and sporting good stores. Look for neoprene or gel cushion models, which do a better job of cushioning — often better than the original inserts that came with your shoes.

Spenco and Dr. Scholl's are two good, easy-to-find brands of inserts.

Cutting Footloose

Specialized relaxation gadgets can provide a welcome vacation for your feet, legs, and back. So many different types of devices are available that it's impossible to mention them all here. In general, they fall into one of two categories: stretchers and massagers.

As people become more aware of how good stretching is for the muscles and how good it feels, more and more gadgets for loosening up the muscles are finding their way on to store shelves. For example, I noticed an ingenious toe-stretching device in one of my walking catalogs the other day: a rubber rectangle with five cutouts. You slip a toe into each hole to get a good stretch and increase circulation. You can use it after you walk to ease toe tension and fatigue or while you walk to keep the Achilles tendon in a stretched position. What will they think of next!

I like stretching gadgets because I don't love to stretch. I find that having some sort of aid makes me more likely to spend those important extra few minutes loosening up my muscles. When you come inside after a walk or turn off your treadmill, your stretching apparatus reminds you to do the right thing.

One of my favorite stretching tools is the Pro Stretch, a $25 piece of plastic shaped like the brake pedal of a car. You place your entire foot on top of it and press your heel down for the single best calf stretch I have ever experienced. Many of my clients agree.

For the back, I like to drape myself over a large plastic ball known as a Physioball or Swiss ball. It gives you a wonderful, safe stretch for the back. You can do dozens of other stretches with the Physioball, too. A company called Flexaball packages a demonstration video with its ball. I love the video, but most people find the Flexaball too small and not as good-quality as some of the other balls on the market.

Several rope and beltlike products are also on the market. I discuss them in detail in the stretching chapter (Chapter 12). I like them because they are simple to use yet very effective if you use them correctly. They're especially good for people with limited flexibility who need some extra help positioning and holding a stretch.

Several types of massagers are available. Some vibrate on the theory that this motion tires out the muscles until they eventually become so exhausted that they relax. Most people I talk to aren't big fans of this type of massager because they feel nothing like the real deal. I've even heard some people complain that, when used near the head and neck, they cause motion sickness.

Other massaging devices thump up and down or massage in a circular pattern. My friend Bob, a licensed massage therapist, had a large thumping device aptly named The Thumper. He tried it out on me one time, and it felt like someone was pounding on my back with a high-powered jackhammer. I was definitely grateful when it stopped.

Still other massagers are simple wooden knobs, stickers, or poles that require a little elbow grease to use.

The Theracane is a large S-shaped rod with a wooden knob on each end. To use it, you place the knob on the area you want to target and use the cane as leverage to work the knob into the muscles. It really goes deep into the muscle; I especially like it for digging into knots along the shoulder blades and back of the thighs.

Getting Help from Walking Aids

I wasn't going to talk about walkers, canes, and other walking aids in this book until my online fitness chat group convinced me otherwise. So many of the people I talk to each week on my one-hour iVillage chat have extolled the virtue of walking aids that I thought they deserve a mention.

Betty Hall, one of my weekly online chatters, calls her 9-pound Pegasus walker her "buddy." Betty has trouble walking because of degenerative disk disease and couldn't get around at all until she got her walker. Like many people I talk to, she was reluctant to use such an obvious walking aid, but after she got over her self-consciousness, she was happy she began using the walker. She now walks a couple of miles in the mall almost every day, something that would not be possible without her buddy.

Using a walking stick or cane may suffice if you don't need quite so much support. Some people even carry them as a personal statement. (Really well-made canes are beautiful.)

After doing a little research, I was amazed to find out that walking canes are much more than a whittled-down stick of wood with a handle. Canes come with two types of handles. The crook-type handle is rounded, and the support-type handle is straight. According to information I received from the House of Canes and Walking Sticks, the support-type handle is preferred 4 to 1. However, the shaft of the cane provides the bulk of the support. For this reason, the shaft of the cane should be solid, not hollow, so that it can bear your weight without cracking, bending, or breaking.

All canes should have rubber tips to prevent slippage. When the tip becomes worn, replace it. Your cane should also have a strap located several inches below the handle so that you can free your hands when you're not walking.

If you're having a great deal of trouble walking, consult with a physician. He may recommend using a walker or cane or perhaps some physical therapy.

A good cane can run you a few hundred bucks, as can a lightweight, sturdy walker. However, if you can't walk without some additional support, consider it money well spent. Check with your insurance carrier; some of them do cover the cost or partial cost of walking aids if prescribed by a medical professional.

Getting Guidance from a Genius

Even though hiring a personal trainer is now more affordable than ever, working with one may still not be a feasible option for you. You may have a crazy lifestyle that prevents you from keeping regular appointments, you may not be able to find a compatible trainer in your area, or you may prefer to work out on your own. Still, there's no substitution for personalized attention.

Enter a product called the Physical Genius Home Trainer, a system that provides a link between you and a personal trainer via the Web.

Here's how this intriguing gadget works: You place the Digital Training Assistant (DTA), a handheld computer unit similar in size and shape to a PalmPilot or a beeper, into a cradle that's attached to your personal computer. With the touch of a button, it links with the Physical Genius Web site. It downloads workout information, such as the duration and intensity of your walk that you have punched in to your DTA, and sends it to your personal trainer. Your personal trainer charts and analyzes the collected data and uploads future workout routines back to you. When you carry the DTA on your walk or to the gym, it guides you through your routine via an easy-to-read digital text display. Besides leading you step by step through your workout, it offers tips on technique and reminders about your goals.

If you currently work with a specific personal trainer some of the time, your trainer can join the Physical Genius trainer's network and continue to train you from a remote location. Or you can let the Physical Genius site assign you a trainer. Your trainer can automatically view and examine your performance and send you instructions, encouragement, adjustments, and messages. She can create a series of graphs and charts that help spot trends in your workouts, weight, and injury patterns.

This nifty system costs $249. The price includes the DTA, software, and access to the Web site. I realize that this invention is a little different from most of the other recommendations I make in this chapter because it's more of a general workout tool rather than something you use exclusively for walking. Still, it can help you improve as a walker because it is a simple way to track your progress and get regular feedback and advice from a fitness expert. You can also use it to track other aspects of your fitness regimen such as weight training, cross-training, and stretching.

Physical Genius is probably the wave of the future. Already an army of copy-cat products is cropping up, though none are yet as sophisticated or advanced in concept. If you are comfortable surfing the Net and punching information into small handheld computer devices, this could be the training gizmo you've been looking for. For more information, check out the Physical Genius Web site at www.physicalgenius.com.

Chapter 19

Ten Great Sources of Walking Information

*W*alking is such a popular activity that you shouldn't have any problems tracking down an abundance of resources on the topic. The trick is to find good, reputable sources. Not every walking and fitness organization has your best interest at heart or is dispensing accurate, up-to-date information. Be very discerning when trying to find out which walking facts and figures to believe and where to spend your money.

The ten sources I've compiled for you are among the best places to seek out ongoing and updated information about walking, health, and fitness in general. I also throw in a few excellent sources for walking clothing and walking gear.

Magazines for Walkers

Walkers are fortunate enough to have *Walking,* a terrific magazine dedicated entirely to them. It offers practical advice, support, and motivation for people interested in a walking-based healthy lifestyle, including current health news, fitness programs, gear and shoe reviews, travel, lowfat recipes, nutrition, and healthful eating. Here's a rundown of the magazine's regular features:

- ✔ **Walking Shorts:** Fitness tips and beauty advice
- ✔ **Nutrition:** The smartest food choices for good health and long life
- ✔ **Active Beauty:** How to make your body look as good as it feels

- ✔ **Walk it Off:** Exercise-based weight-loss strategies
- ✔ **Health:** The art and science of staying well
- ✔ **Walking Gear:** The best in walking apparel and accessories
- ✔ **Training Guide:** Secrets from trainers and fitness experts
- ✔ **The Great Outdoors:** The best vacation destinations for walkers
- ✔ **Spotlight**: Real-life walking heroes share their stories

Walking also publishes a weight-loss newsletter, Walk Off Weight, and a free Walking Tip Sheet, an information-packed card that you can tack to your refrigerator. It is a handy reference on how to build a walking program and offers tips on selecting shoes, walking in an event, proper walking technique, and stretching exercises. The magazine has a national network of walking clubs of all types as well as reviews on other walking resources and publications. Contact information for *Walking* is located in the appendix.

Although *Walking* is the only large national publication geared exclusively for walkers, dozens of other fitness magazines provide interesting and accurate information on walking and general fitness. I recommend giving at least some of them an occasional read. Here's a list of a few magazines that frequently offer useful walking, fitness, exercise, and health articles:

- ✔ *Shape*
- ✔ *Fitness*
- ✔ *Prevention*
- ✔ *American Health*
- ✔ *Men's Health*
- ✔ *Men's Fitness*
- ✔ *Cooking Light*
- ✔ *Family Circle*
- ✔ *Redbook*

Web Sites Worth Visiting

An astonishing abundance of walking and other health sources is available on the Internet. Trouble is, you have no way to tell who is putting that information out there and how accurate it is. For example, one site that I looked at advocated walking in bare feet — even on city streets.

Much of what's on the Net is designed to get you to spend your money. For example, Rockport shoes has an excellent Web site chock-full of great walking tips and motivational advice. It is also laced with ads and gives you plenty of opportunities to order its shoes. I'm not saying that there's anything wrong with a healthy dose of capitalism — just maintain an awareness of where you're clicking your mouse.

Be especially careful about FAQ (Frequently Asked Question) pages. Although some are carefully researched and well executed, anyone can slap together his own walking and fitness site. I have found the accuracy of this type of information to be a little spotty. I don't want to say that there aren't any good ones. But I do recommend sticking to FAQs put together by well-known, reputable organizations like the American Council on Exercise and the American College of Sports Medicine or by individuals who have the education, experience, and certification credentials to speak with authority.

The Internet is still new and growing faster than the speed of a race walker. New sites come and go every hour of every day. I've compiled a list of some stable-for-the-moment URLs (Web addresses) that I think are worth a visit.

Walking URLs

If you're looking for specific information on walking, these sites are a good place to start.

About.com

This Web site, at `http://walking.miningco.com/`, offers excellent information about walking and other health and fitness topics. It has more than 100 archived walking articles as well as walking programs for all levels, reviews of walking shoes, and links to dozens of other walking sites. Plenty of merchandise is also for sale here, so be prepared to be bombarded with ads and admonishments to buy, buy, buy.

The Walking Connection

This site, at `www.walkingconnection.com/Walk_Members_Home_Page.html`, is dedicated to those who love to walk, hike, and go on walking vacations. You can join the Walking Connection Club and receive automatic notifications about events as well as the club's free hard-copy or online publications. This is an extensive resource for information, products, and services geared specifically to walkers.

Women.com Walking Clubs

A good site for experienced and novice walkers alike is `www.women.com/clubs/walking.html`. Regular features include Walk Talk, a Q&A column, and Footnotes, an advice column. The site also has a chat and message board where you can communicate with other walkers from around the globe.

Racewalk.com

Take a look at the official Web site of the USA Track and Field Association, www.racewalk.com. It provides information on starting and improving your walking program for both competitive and noncompetitive walkers. It offers guidance on gathering free and at-cost walking resources and gear. Purchases you make through the site help support U.S. track athletes.

General fitness URLs

Check out these Web sites for information on general fitness.

Health World

Set up like a college campus, this site, at www.healthy.net, offers you everything from words of wisdom from top experts to a free Medline-published research search. It is easy to navigate, and information is updated frequently.

American Volkssport Association

Volkssport is a noun of German derivation that means a group of "people's" sports including walking, swimming, skiing, snowshoeing, and biking. The verb *volkssporting* means to participate in those sports. A *volksmarch* is a walking event, sometimes also called a *volkswalk*.

In Germany, these events were originally termed volkswanderung — "volkswandering." Reportedly, this word was difficult for American World War II military personnel stationed in Germany to understand, so they started using the term volksmarsch. The word eventually evolved into "volksmarch" in the United States.

Thousands of volkssport clubs have sprung up around the world, allied together as the International Volkssport Federation. As a national division of the IVF, the American Volkssport Association promotes noncompetitive walking events for everyone. More than 500 volkssport clubs have been organized in the U.S.

Clubs host weekend events in which members select interesting trails and walking routes for everyone to enjoy. Club members make their trail selections based on safety, scenic interest, historic areas, natural beauty, and walkability. They then invite the community to come and enjoy it on a weekend or a weekday evening. Most volksmarches are held as noncompetitive 6-mile (10-kilometer) walks. These events are not races, and you don't have to collect pledges. Instead they are meant to be something that you can do for fun and fitness.

Club dues are usually minimal, often less than $10 per year. Volkswalk events are a great way to meet other active walkers in your area. Clubs welcome new members, but you don't have to join a club to enjoy the volksmarch events. To find out more about forming a club, contact the American Volkssport Association. For contact information, turn to the appendix.

Fitness Partner Connection

Check out www.primusweb.com/fitnesspartner if you're looking for a "jump" site with links to almost a hundred other fitness sites. It is jam-packed with articles on cooking and nutrition, training, mental fitness, sports medicine, and lots more. I especially love the Activity Calculator, which tells you the number of calories your body burns while doing 158 activities in the gym, at home, while training, during your daily life, and when you're on the job.

The American Council on Exercise

ACE is the largest personal trainer certifying body in the world and is well respected in the fitness industry. Visit the official ACE Web site, at www.acefitness.org, and you'll find information on how to become certified, find a certified trainer, and evaluate a certified trainer. The site contains a lot more information, too, on everything from fitness tips to lowfat cooking advice.

FitnessLink

"All the News that's Fit" is the tagline at this Web site, located at www.fitness link.com/index.html. And indeed, a new health story is posted daily. You can also find an archive of the latest reputable health information, facts, and opinions. This is also an excellent jump site to other fitness pages on the Web.

iVillage

Visit iVillage, at www.ivillage.com, to see one of the few sites on the Net geared toward women. Its fitness and beauty pages are particularly well done. I write for its Fit By Friday column, which deals with starting a fitness program and staying motivated. Other iVillage fitness highlights include the Walking Club, the Chub Club, and the Community Shape Up Challenge. You'll find columns, boards, and chats on any health and fitness topic you can think of, all of them written and monitored by top professionals. If you don't see anything that suits you, you can request permission to start a new club.

Your Local Mall

The Meadow Glen Mall in Medford, Massachusetts, sponsors the excellent Mall Walkers Club run in conjunction with Lawrence Memorial Hospital. Participation is free of charge to anyone interested. Each day, the mall opens its doors to registered mall walkers two hours before the stores open. Walkers follow a 1-mile route of three trips around the inside of the mall. The mall personnel keep track of their mileage for them, and mall walkers receive prizes when they hit different milestones.

The Coronado Mall Walkers Club in Albuquerque, New Mexico, has a similar program. So do the Hanes Mall in Winston-Salem, North Carolina, and the Miracle City Mall in Titusville, Florida. The Oxford Valley Mall Walkers Club in Langhorne, Pennsylvania, opens its doors at 7 a.m. and boasts a strong base of 1,700 members.

According to the National Organization of Mall Walkers, more than 1,000 malls across the country have official mall walkers clubs. Many others have informal walking groups. Consider joining one for days when the weather is bad or if you live in an area where safety is a concern. Mall walking is great if you're just starting out, too. Malls offer plenty of places to stop and rest along the way, and it's also pretty hard to get lost — just head toward Old Navy and take a left.

Check with the information or customer service desk at your local mall for information about its walking club. Many malls provide maps, offer prizes, and set up walking buddy programs free of charge. A local hospital, YMCA, or fitness center often works in conjunction with the mall to set up walking clinics and monitor the mall walking programs. Some malls hold walking events and competitions as well.

The Government

Looking for a great place to hike? Check with your local parks and recreation department. Interested in retracing the steps of your city's founding forefathers? Ask your local historical society for a map and find out when it gives guided walking tours. Many national, state, and local government agencies are a great source of information for creative and offbeat walking venues.

I like to hike the trails in upstate New York. A few years ago, I wrote to the local parks and recreation department, which sent me trail maps, tips for winter and summer hiking, and a pamphlet on safe hiking — all free of charge. Even though I have been trekking around that area most of my life, I discovered new trails and learned a lot of interesting details about the local history, flora, and fauna from the information I received.

Even the U.S. Department of Transportation has gotten into the act. It actually considers walking a form of transportation — imagine that! The agency provides information packets on how people can make their community a more walkable place. For instance, it has developed the Pedestrian Safety Roadshow, a program aimed at identifying and solving the potential problems that affect pedestrian safety.

Another example of a government sponsored walking program is Shape Up America! This is an organization of the Partnership for a Walkable America along with the National Safety Council, the U.S. Department of Transportation, the Centers for Disease Control and Prevention, and other organizations from the nonprofit, governmental, and commercial sectors. The mission of the partnership is to increase awareness of the healthful benefits of walking and to increase the safety and accessibility of sidewalks and pedestrian pathways for walking in communities throughout the United States.

The first thing to do if you are interested in government-sponsored walking events, resources, and programs is flip through your telephone directory's yellow pages. Most have a section of government agency listings, along with brief descriptions of the types of services and information they offer. Don't forget to check Web sites, too. For example, the Spokane Parks and Recreation Department has links to all of its walking and hiking events on its home page.

The URL `famnet.com/govern.htm` lists many national government agencies. You can skim through this list to find the agency you are interested in. Various government departments — from the President's Council on Physical Fitness to the U.S. Fish and Wildlife Service — have walking tidbits to offer you. I particularly like Parknet, a national information registry of parks and landmarks. It lists dozens of nature hikes and large-city landmark walking tours, great ideas for vacations, and walking getaways.

TOPS Club, Inc.

TOPS Club, Inc. (Take Off Pounds Sensibly) was established as a nonprofit organization in 1948 and today has nearly 300,000 members and 11,700 chapters worldwide. In 1997, TOPS launched the largest ongoing community-based walking program in North America. The TOPS Walking Program reflects the organization's commitment to the health-enhancing benefits of walking. The program has been designed to provide information and materials that can easily be adapted to fit the specific needs of individuals and groups throughout the United States.

The thing I like best about TOPS is that, unlike many other major weight loss organizations, it has nothing to sell in the way of prepackaged meals or diet supplements. When you join TOPS, you are truly joining a support group to help you lose weight and begin a shape-up program. TOPS often works in conjunction with local physicians or helps you take the advice of your personal physician and put it into an action plan.

Members meet weekly in their local chapters for a private weigh-in followed by a program. Programs vary but all in some way provide members with positive reinforcement and motivation in adhering to their food and exercise plans. Many follow the walking program designed by the national TOPS chapter. Other benefits of membership include a Nutrition Monograph for Taking Off Pounds Sensibly; a TOPS-sponsored book containing the exchange system for meal planning, as well as practical advice on nutrition; TOPS retreats, rallies, and recognition days; and a monthly membership magazine.

TOPS club fees are $20 in the U.S. and $25 in Canada. The fee includes participation in the walking program and all the other club offerings. To obtain more information about TOPS and a free brochure about the TOPS Walking Program, see the contact information in the appendix.

Travel Clubs

Nothing is more frustrating than getting into a good walking and weight loss routine only to fall off the wagon when you travel or go on vacation. Most people complain about gaining weight or not getting enough exercise when they travel. Why not combine walking with pleasure and take a vacation that purposely involves a lot of walking?

Sit down with your travel agent and explain the type of trip you want to take. Let her know that you would like it to be as active a trip as possible. The possibilities are endless. You can take a trekking trip, as my husband and I often do, through a national or international park. If you're not into roughing it, try a walking tour through Europe or a major U.S. city. New York City offers all types of walking tours with different focuses. You can take a walking tour of museums, of national monuments, or even of infamous crime scenes if you're so inclined.

Most major cities offer the same types of tours. D.C. Walking Tours, based in the nation's capital, leads tours through beautiful gardens, trendy neighborhoods, and historical homes and landmarks at a nominal cost.

The following travel organizations provide extensive information on walking travel. They offer prepackaged walking tours to anywhere in the world, from Poland to the North Pole.

✔ **The Friendly Trails Travel Club:** This is a leisure walkers travel club dedicated to finding comfortable vacations for its members at the lowest possible price. These vacations can be arranged so that nonwalkers can enjoy themselves while more active vacationers participate in the walks. The club is affiliated with the American Hiking Society (AHS), American Volkssport Association (AVA), and the International Leisure Walkers Association (ILWA).

✔ **American Discovery Trail:** The American Discovery Trail is America's first coast-to-coast hiking, biking, and equestrian trail. It passes through metropolitan areas like San Francisco, Denver, Cincinnati, and Washington, D.C.; traces numerous pioneer trails; leads to 14 national parks and 16 national forests; and visits more than 10,000 historical, cultural, and natural sites of significance! This 6,356-mile trail is itself a national landmark in the making — one that provides weekend getaways, family fun, real adventure opportunities, and a taste of true Americana. Contact the ADT for a state-by-state look at what's offered to hikers and walkers throughout the U.S.

- ✔ **European Ramblers Association (ERA):** Founded in 1969, the European Ramblers Association is a federation, currently based in Germany, of 56 walking organizations from 27 European countries. Contact it for European walking vacations and maps of European footpaths.

- ✔ **Backroads:** This travel organization offers biking, walking, hiking, and multisport vacations all over North America, Europe, Asia, the Pacific, South America, and Africa. The number one active travel agency in the world, it offers all types of trips for all budgets, tastes, ages, and abilities. First-class hotel accommodations, gourmet dining, van-trailer support, and professional trip leaders are some of the special features. You can choose from inn and camping trips ranging from 2 to 15 days.

- ✔ **Specialty Travel Index ONLINE:** This is a directory of walking and adventure vacations around the world. As you look through the Internet version of this magazine, you'll find detailed information about thousands of both exotic and straightforward vacations, offered by more than 600 tour operators and outfitters around the globe.

All contact information about these groups is located in the appendix. You can research these as well as other walking travel sources and then bring them to your travel agent. She can then fine-tune and personalize your trip as well as make all your travel arrangements.

If the resources in this section don't seem to fit into the type of trip you'd like to take, do a Web search. If you enter the location you are interested in visiting and the word "walking," you should come up with information about a walking or hiking tour of that area. For example, if you are interested in walking through Ireland, enter *Ireland and walking* into your search engine. I did this and came away with more than two dozen excellent leads to take to my travel agent.

A Personal Trainer

At some point, you may want to consider hiring a personal trainer to look over your walking and exercise program. She can offer you information on everything from how to correct your walking posture to the safest way to increase your mileage and intensity.

A personal trainer can help you attain your goals faster, teach you new exercises, provide you with current exercise information, and correct your mistakes. The best time to hire a trainer is when you're first starting out, after a long layoff, or if you're stuck in a rut. A personal trainer need not be a long-term commitment, either: Provided that you have chosen an experienced and knowledgeable trainer, a few sessions are often all you need to get on the right track.

Depending on what part of the country you live in, personal training fees run anywhere from $35 to $200 a session. I recommend asking someone you trust and respect for a recommendation and then interviewing the trainer before you hire somone. Ask for a trial session before committing to a larger block of time. In order to maximize your time, come armed with all the information you want to cover and the goals you want to achieve.

Before you fork over your money to a personal trainer, evaluate her based on the following criteria:

✔ **Certification:** A certification shows that your trainer has at least made a commitment to study for a few weeks and has demonstrated a minimum level of knowledge. However, not all certifications are equal. Although neither a national certification program nor any legal guidelines have been established for personal trainers, here are several generally accepted and well-respected certifications:

- American College of Sports Medicine.

- American Council on Exercise.

- National Strength and Conditioning Association.

- Aerobics and Fitness Association of America. Note: This is the only national certification that offers a special certification course in walking.

- National Academy of Sports Medicine.

These aren't the only legitimate certifications. Many colleges and universities offer their own extensive certification programs, and some health clubs put their employees through rigorous training courses. Ask to see a copy of each actual certificate when you are hiring a trainer.

✔ **Education:** A degree means that your trainer went through four years of undergraduate work or did two to three years of graduate work to study all sorts of topics related to exercise and health. Degrees to look for are exercise physiology, exercise science, physical therapy, occupational therapy, fitness management, sports medicine, physical education, and kinesiology.

In recent years, registered nurses, physical therapists, massage therapists, and even physicians are getting into the personal training game. If your trainer has one of these advanced degrees, it's a real plus; these trainers sometimes can accept insurance reimbursement if a doctor prescribes your sessions.

✔ **Experience:** Chose a trainer who has had at least two years of experience, preferably at a reputable health club. All the certifications and education in the world are no substitute for a large dose of practical knowledge.

✔ **Liability insurance:** In this day and age, it is important for a personal trainer to carry liability insurance. This protects both you and the trainer in case you get hurt during the course of your training sessions. Ask to see the most up-to-date insurance certificate and information. It's a smart idea to keep a copy in your files as well.

Catalogs

When you're looking for the perfect walking parka or searching for the best bargain on walking shoes, sometimes mall and department store shopping just doesn't cut it. Dozens of specialty catalogs carry hard-to-locate walking products. And this is one time when it's okay to sit back and let your fingers do the walking.

Let me share my list of preferred walking specialty catalogs with you. (Turn to the appendix for contact information.) Some of these are my best-kept secrets, so don't tell anyone.

✔ **Road Runner Sports:** Okay, forget that the name has the word "runner" in it — this is a great source of walking clothes and shoes. The prices are lower than what you'll find in the store, and the phone operators are extremely knowledgeable. It runs great sales on discontinued shoe models and even has a notification service to give you updates as to the availability of your favorite products. Join its Run America Club to receive further discounts, a newsletter, and other benefits.

✔ **Title Nine Sports:** This catalog carries walking and other sports gear and clothing designed especially for women. In particular, it carries the brands Moving Comfort and In Sport, two labels that specialize in women's clothing. I have a Moving Comfort windbreaker that all my friends covet — it's extra long in the back so it covers my butt.

✔ **Health for Life:** This catalog is a good source for training books and gadgets.

✔ **Patagonia:** Patagonia has long been considered one of the highest-quality designers of hiking, walking, and camping gear. Although its products are on the pricey side, they are well made and last for years, so they are an excellent value. It specializes in fleeces, parkas, and wool clothing. I often buy Patagonia products as baby gifts, especially for my friend Katie's children, who brave the winters in Minneapolis.

✔ **Collage Video:** This complete guide to exercise videos offers all sorts of exercise videos, including how-to walking technique videos. Collage also sells audiotapes that you can listen to while you walk. Trained video consultants who have tried every single product offered in the catalog answer the phones and are happy to share their opinions.

Other Walkers

Jeanie, a client of mine who does a lot of walking, was the first to tell me about a new walking and running path that opened in New York on the Lower East Side. The path is in a direction I rarely headed, so I may not have stumbled on to it for months. Now it's one of my favorite places to walk and run. Jeanie also clued me in on the location of some little-known bathrooms and water fountains along the route as well.

This sort of thing happens to me all the time. I gather all sorts of interesting information from other walkers. You, too, should keep your ears open and listen to what other walkers have to say. You just might learn a thing or two.

Of course, you have to be ready to evaluate any and all information to separate old wives' tales from fact. I've had people offer me advice on everything from bogus weight loss treatments to walking shoes for my dog. Just because someone tells you something doesn't mean that you should put your common sense on the shelf. If it sounds too wacky to be true, it probably is.

The best place to find other walkers to listen to is through your local walking club. If your town doesn't have one, it probably has a running club, which very often includes a walkers group. You can also hang out where other walkers walk, like the park, the mall, your church, or fitness center. I know many people who have formed very successful walking groups at work.

If you have trouble finding other walkers to walk and talk with locally, you can always find them on the Net. Dozens of chat rooms are dedicated to walkers. The Walking Club at iVillage.com is just one example. Walkers of all ages and levels from all over the world come together to discuss their favorite pastime.

Congregating with other walkers is a good way to stay motivated. Besides offering each other tips and advice, we offer each other motivation and support. A woman who once came to my iVillage Fit By Friday chat was very depressed and discouraged because she couldn't get her fitness program into gear. Thanks to the encouragement and enthusiasm of the other participants, she lost about ten pounds and is walking three times a week for up to 30 minutes at a time.

Chapter 20

Ten Ways to Stay Motivated

● ●

In This Chapter

▶ Deciding on a goal or destination

▶ Enjoying music, TV, books, or the Net

▶ Exercising with a human or canine buddy

▶ Giving yourself a reward

▶ Walking for competition or a cause

● ●

My family always considered my mother fitness-proof even though my father is a cardiologist and I've been in the exercise business as a personal trainer, exercise physiologist, and corporate fitness consultant for more than 15 years.

Over the years we tried many tactics to get my mom to focus on her health. We bought her a gym membership. She used it only once, even though the gym is less than a block away from work. Another time we bought her a cross-country ski machine for the TV room. Within a month, it officially became a clothes hanger. She resisted every single effort by anyone to help her get into shape.

Everything changed in 1998 when an editor from *Good Housekeeping* magazine approached me about doing a fitness makeover on someone. I asked her if I could use my mom, and she said yes. I didn't think my mother would agree to it, but to my surprise, she did. And so Operation Mom began.

Charlie Cherney, an old friend and personal trainer who lives in my hometown of Kingston, New York, conducted Operation Mom. Charlie got my mother walking on the treadmill three to five times a week and weight training two to three times a week. He scheduled several appointments for her with a registered dietitian who completely overhauled my mother's diet and eating habits.

Over the next few months, my mother showed up for every single training session. She started out barely able to walk for 10 minutes at an easy pace. However, after a few months, she was walking 2 miles on a slight incline at a respectable 15-minutes-per-mile clip. She made significant improvements in her strength and flexibility, too. By the time we took the "after" pictures for the magazine, she was hooked on walking as a way of life, had lost 45 pounds, and had finally kicked her two-pack-a-day smoking habit. It is truly an amazing transformation. I am eternally indebted to *Good Housekeeping* for allowing me to pull off Operation Mom.

The threat of her picture in a national magazine, which has 27 million readers, was the motivation my mother needed to get herself into shape. Admittedly, not everyone has an opportunity like that. But my point is, you need to find something to inspire you to lace up your walking shoes and head out the door each day. This chapter contains several suggestions that can help keep you pumped about your walking and fitness program.

Reach for a Goal

In Chapter 2, I tell you everything you need to know about setting goals for your walking program. Have you gone through the goal-setting process yet? If not, I strongly suggest that you do. Smart and thoughtful goal setting is one of the keys to success.

Goal setting is important because it gives a purpose and a shape to your program. I find it tough to get energized about my workouts if they are aimless. For me, nothing is worse than facing the treadmill and thinking, "Okay, what am I going to do with you today?" Many of my clients tell me the same thing.

One of my clients has had a weight problem all her life. She has always had trouble staying motivated for long periods of time. When she first came to me, I gave her a preliminary fitness evaluation and then explained the results of each test. Together we came up with some decisive fitness goals for her by using the principles outlined in Chapter 2. Instead of using body weight as a measure of success, we decided to focus on a four-point drop in body fat percentage and an improvement in her cardiovascular fitness ranking from poor to average. To achieve these objectives, we set up a 4-day-a-week program that fit into her busy schedule. She walked on the treadmill for 30 minutes and did a series of stretches and weight training exercises each day. At her three-month evaluation, the news was good: She dropped two body-fat percentage points and scored average for cardiovascular conditioning. Her revised goals include dropping another 2 percent of body fat and ranking good in cardiovascular conditioning.

I include two goal-setting tools in this book:

> ✔ **Your personal testing scorecard:** Use this chart, which you can find at the end of Chapter 1, to write down and keep track of your current level of fitness. This chart also includes the ideal scores for you to work toward.

✔ **Goal-setting worksheet:** Use this worksheet (see Chapter 2) as a step-by-step goal and program planner. I recommend making copies of this sheet so that you can reuse it whenever you want to reevaluate the purpose of your walking program.

Write It Down

Keeping a workout and diet diary charts what you have accomplished on a day-to-day basis. When you flip through your diary, you can easily spot trends. If your program is successful, then you have a written record of what it took to achieve your accomplishments. If you're not successful, you can use your diary to determine why.

A workout diary also keeps you honest. You can't cry about not losing weight if your diary tells you that you eat three doughnuts every Tuesday and Thursday night before you go to sleep or you haven't done any exercise in several weeks. In fact, the act of writing things down can, in and of itself, be a powerful motivator. If you don't want to write down that you ate those three doughnuts, perhaps you won't eat them!

Include as much information in your workout and eating diary as you think is necessary. The more detail you include, the better. For example, I have one client who writes down her mealtime moods. This type of record keeping is a bit much for me, but she tells me that it helps her avoid overeating when she is upset or stressed.

Here are some types of information that you may want to include in your workout and diet diary:

✔ **Walking information:** Workout time, distance, heart rate, intensity (including your rating of perceived exertion and how you felt overall), walking route, time of walk, weather conditions, injuries, aches, and pains. You also can include any suggestions for improvement.

✔ **General fitness information:** Exercises performed, number of sets and repetitions, your weight, exercise intensity, and notes for improvement.

✔ **Nutrition and diet information:** Foods eaten, portion size, time of meals, satisfaction rating, and notes for improvement.

You can reproduce the Walker's Log in Chapter 2 and use it as your workout and diet diary. You can also purchase a fancy workout log; dozens of hard copy and computerized logs are on the market. Or you can simply use a blank notebook as your diary. I created my own log as a Word document on my computer.

Entertain Yourself

Finding a way to keep yourself entertained while you're walking on the treadmill can be a pleasant diversion, one that keeps boredom at bay and keeps you coming back for your workout day after day. Why not consider watching television or listening to music or the latest best-seller while you're walking?

Use headphones or a personal stereo only when you are walking on a treadmill or another place that is very safe. I do not recommend listening to headphones while you are out walking on the street, on a trail, or by the side of a road. Doing so distracts you from your surroundings. You may not hear a car coming or someone sneaking up behind you. All your senses must be working at full capacity whenever you walk outside. Safety must always come before entertainment.

Watching TV

Planning your treadmill workout to coincide with your favorite TV show is a good way to combine the two activities. You can keep up with the story line without flopping on the couch and inhaling a bag of potato chips. Plus, treadmill walking while watching TV makes the time fly by.

One of our gyms is always packed at 1 p.m. because everyone comes in to see what Erica Kane is up to on *All My Children*. (By the way, it's not just women who are watching.) "I can get my workout in and visit Pine Valley at the same time," one soap opera viewer once confided to me.

If you like the idea of watching the tube while on the treadmill, join a gym that has TV access. Some gyms have "cardio theaters" that allow members to plug their headphones into any one of several TV sets. Because there is no external sound, those who want to watch can do so without disturbing those who don't. I belong to one gym that has an extensive cardio theater. This gym is open 24 hours a day, so I can pop in and get a workout while I watch the 11 p.m. rerun of a *Seinfeld* episode. Many of the treadmills are usually taken at that time by people who do the same.

Here's one caveat about watching TV while treadmill walking: Don't get too involved in your soap opera or sitcom or you risk taking a tumble. Stay within an arm's reach of the handrails. If you're particularly clumsy, you may want to hold on to the rails lightly as you watch TV — you don't need to grasp the rails too hard.

Listening to music

Listening to music is a great way to stay motivated. Instead of listening to the radio, as many people do, I make my own personal tape compilations every few months or so. That way, I hear only the songs I like, with no commercial interruptions.

You can purchase tapes made especially for walking. Two Web sites, amazon.com and cdnow.com, sell preprogrammed tapes developed especially for working out. These tapes have music tempo changes that correspond to each phase of your workout. One treadmill, the CD Coach by Icon Fitness, even has a built-in CD player. You can purchase special workout CDs for this treadmill that automatically change the pace and incline of the treadmill to match the cadence of the music. I tried this treadmill at a trade show, and though I wasn't impressed with the quality of the machine itself, I thought the CD technology was absolutely amazing.

Enjoying books on tape

Catching up on your reading with books on tape may be a good deal if you're short on time. You may find this a more motivating strategy than listening to music or watching TV. Virtually every book now has an audio version — even *Fitness For Dummies,* which was read aloud by my co-author, Suzanne Schlosberg. Famous actors and actresses, including Meryl Streep, Brad Pitt, and Alan Arkin, often lend their voices to their favorite books. Perhaps your gym even has a books-on-tape club.

In 1998, several literary groups published lists of the best English-speaking novels of the last 100 years. Several of my clients formed a books-on-tape club; they purchase books on tape that are on one of the top 100 lists and trade them with each other. They are slowly working their way through each novel and hope to listen to every book on the list within 24 months.

Surfing the Net while You Walk

Health clubs have long featured sound systems, big-screen televisions, and racks of reading material as a convenience for their members. But clubs have introduced new equipment to make cardiovascular multitasking even easier. Computerized "exertainment" stations, which come attached to treadmills as well as stair steppers and stationary bikes, are the latest gizmos that aim to keep people exercising. With a light tap on the touch screen, you can surf the Net, check your e-mail, read the paper, watch TV, listen to a CD, do some research for a project at work — or do all at the same time — as long as you keep moving. If you stop exercising, the default screen politely prods, "Please resume exercising."

Look for one of these set-ups coming soon to a gym near you. Net Pulse, E-Zone, and IFE (Interactive Fitness Environment) are three companies that manufacture these systems.

Think!

Put on your thinking cap to solve a problem, come up with new ideas, or make plans. This is a good motivational tip for people who don't like watching *ER* reruns as a means of escape. When I walk, I like to think about things I am writing about. I can outline entire books and articles in my head while I walk.

Just don't think too hard. You always want to stay aware of your surroundings. I have one client who walked off a bridge because he was so engrossed in his thoughts. Fortunately, he wasn't hurt. And one time I was walking around lost in thought when I walked smack into a no-parking sign. Of course, several people I knew just happened to witness this embarrassing event.

Don't think about such serious or stressful topics that you don't feel relaxed. For this reason, you may want to think about pleasant things. My friend Burt always thinks about a trip he took to New Orleans as a teenager.

Find a Buddy

Some people find it hard to stay motivated when they work out alone. You may find that if you make a date to walk with a friend, you're a lot less likely to break it than if you walk alone. But if your friend doesn't show up, go anyway.

If you can't find a friend or family member to walk with, consider joining a formal club or walking group. Check your yellow pages or the Net for a TOPS (Take Off Pounds Sensibly) walking group or a volkssports walking group. Each of these organizations has hundreds of chapters throughout the country and the rest of the world. If you can't find a walking group listed in your area, check with a local running club, which often has a walking section within its ranks.

Some walking clubs have buddy bulletin boards. One such board is located at the New York Road Runners club on the Upper East Side in Manhattan. You can post your walking or running pace, preferred walking time, and the area where you'd like to walk. Then you simply wait for someone looking for a similar situation to come along and respond. Many clubs prescreen the boards to weed out the weirdos and whackos.

Consider hooking up with a virtual walking buddy. Dozens of walking support groups, chats, and bulletin boards are located on the Net. I once put two walking buddies in touch via e-mail. Both were having similar problems staying motivated about their workouts. Now they e-mail each other daily to discuss their workouts and offer words of encouragement and advice. One lives in Kansas, and the other lives in New Jersey. They've never met personally — and probably never will — yet they've helped each other tremendously. You gotta love technology.

Walking with Fido

Walking buddies don't have to be human. Millions of dog owners walk their dogs at least twice a day. If you own a dog, you have a ready, willing, and able walking partner. But keep in mind that, though most dogs make eager walking companions, they don't walk to get in shape, so they may have a different agenda than you do. Here are some tips to make exercising with your pup an enjoyable experience for both of you:

- ✔ Precede each workout with a 5- to 10-minute walk to let him relieve himself and mark his territory. You can use this as your warm-up.

- ✔ Obey all leash laws. That means honoring all pooper-scooper laws as well.

- ✔ If your dog constantly stops to sniff and inspect, give a firm but gentle tug on the leash. After a while, he'll bypass all but the most irresistible sights and scents. If he absolutely must stop to check something out, cut him some slack.

- ✔ When walking on or alongside a road, face traffic and train your dog to stay on your left side so you don't interfere with traffic flow. Teach him the heel command so that he doesn't charge across busy intersections.

- ✔ Bring along plenty of water for your dog to drink, especially on hot days. I taught my greyhound, Zoomer, to drink from a water bottle, but it took me a few months to get him to do it. Recently I purchased a product at the neighborhood pet store for about $6 called Handi-Drink. It's a water bottle with a trough attachment. When your dog is thirsty, you simply pour water into the trough, and the dog can lap it up.

Have a Destination

If you are the type of person who just doesn't understand why anyone would want to walk aimlessly around the neighborhood, walk in circles around a track, or, worst of all, walk nowhere on a treadmill, try choosing a destination. Having somewhere to walk to or from can give you a sense of purpose. Here are some suggested destinations:

- ✓ **Work:** If it's too far to walk the whole way to your job, consider getting off the train or bus one stop earlier or walking one train or bus stop farther. I walk a mile to and from work every day, sometimes several times a day.

- ✓ **The store:** You can walk to and from the corner store, the mall, or the shopping center provided they are close enough and aren't along a major highway that is unsafe for pedestrians. If one way is enough for you, arrange to have someone pick you up for the return trip. Carry a knapsack or pull a cart to carry your purchases.

- ✓ **The gym:** Incorporate your walk to and from your fitness facility into your workout.

- ✓ **A friend's house:** You can hang out for a while and ask your friend to drive you back home or bribe your kids to pick you up. Or, if it's a nice day, ask your friend to walk you home.

- ✓ **Lunch or dinner:** Walk to the nearest restaurant or pick up your food instead of having it delivered. You'll burn off some of the calories contained in the meal.

- ✓ **Your kids' school:** Meet your children after school, at the playground, or at their bus stop. You can spend a little bonding time with them and get your walk in. Of course, this idea usually doesn't work with teenagers.

Walk in a Nice Place

Whenever possible, choose a walking route where you can enjoy the scenery and soak up the sites. Pleasant and enjoyable surroundings are always more motivating than surroundings that are boring and dreary. Once when I was on a business trip to Dallas, I had to walk through an industrial area. I found it so disheartening that I cut my workout short.

If you live in a city, try to plan your walks so that you hit a park, some gardens, or some interesting sights. I know a woman who used to walk uptown on a path along the Hudson River in lower Manhattan each day. She began to find it very discouraging, and when I asked her why, she said that giant skyscrapers and gaudy corporate logos affixed to buildings were all she saw. One large neon umbrella logo particularly bummed her out; she said it seemed to cast a bad mood over her entire walk. I recommended that she head in the opposite direction so that she could avoid the dreaded umbrella and instead enjoy a view of the Statue of Liberty for almost the entire workout. She reports that she now walks with more pep in her step.

Consider planning a trip to a place with beautiful places to walk. This advice can help you keep in shape while you travel. If you walk on a treadmill, you can purchase videotapes that simulate walking through some beautiful parts of the world. The other day I took a stroll on a Hawaiian beach without leaving the health club.

Reward Yourself

You give your kids five bucks when they bring home good grades on their report card. You give your golden retriever a doggy treat when he fetches the Frisbee. You have to be nice to yourself, too. Rewarding yourself for a job well done can be fun and inspiring.

You can reward yourself for both short-term and long-term goals. If you make it through an entire 45-minute walk without stopping once, treat yourself to new pair of walking socks. If you get through the entire week without missing a workout, rent that movie you've been dying to see on Friday night. If you finally reach your body fat percent goal, buy yourself a new outfit.

Just make sure that your rewards are not counterproductive. For instance, I don't recommend using food as a reward. You don't want to blow a whole walk's worth of calories during dessert. But who am I to say? If eating is what motivates you, you can use food as a reward as long as you keep it in perspective and dole out the edible treats wisely.

Make your goals creative and meaningful. They don't necessarily have to cost anything either. I know one guy whose wife got into the act. She told him that if he'd stick with his program for one month, she'd take out the garbage for a week. He did and she did.

Compete

Sprinting across a finish line is a very satisfying feeling, even if you're not the one who breaks the tape. If competition appeals to you, consider entering some local road races and training to compete in them. Training for a competition is a great way to give structure and purpose to your workout routine. It can inspire you to try new techniques and work out harder.

Few communities offer races specifically for walkers, but in most cities, you can find races that include divisions for both runners and walkers. Sometimes the events also include a race walk division. If you can't find a walking competition, consider entering a running event and racing against the clock. Many people, for instance, walk the New York and Chicago Marathons instead of running them. Check your newspaper, athletic apparel stores, or running club Web sites for information on races.

Fighting a crowd of walkers and runners may not appeal to you, but that doesn't mean you can't get in the competitive spirit. Try doing a time trial every week or so and aiming for a personal best. For instance, you may want to better your time for a 1-mile walk or improve upon your fastest 2-mile time when you're walking up a 2 percent incline on the treadmill. If you record your various time trials, you'll be amazed at how much you improve over the course of a few weeks.

Competition isn't for everyone. You either like it or you don't. But if you do like it, training for and competing in races can be one of the most motivating experiences you'll ever have.

Walk for a Cause

Nearly every important cause holds a yearly walkathon to raise money for research and to increase awareness. You may feel that your walking program is more meaningful if you train to complete one of these charitable events.

I once participated in a Save the Children 6-hour relay event to raise money for starving children all over the world. I got my friends, family, and coworkers to pledge anywhere from a nickel to a dollar per mile. I managed to run-walk 32 miles in 6 hours and raise thousands of dollars. Although I was tired at the end of the event, I had a deep sense of satisfaction because I had made a positive contribution to a worthwhile cause.

If you are interested in walking for a cause, check your local newspaper listings. Walkathons benefit such excellent causes as breast cancer, AIDS, Alzheimer's disease, diabetes, and multiple sclerosis.

If you have an interest in raising money for a particular group, contact the organization directly to find out what events it has planned for the upcoming months. You can build your entire training schedule around participation. If no event is planned in the near future for your immediate area, you may want to consider traveling to participate in one elsewhere or starting one of your own. In either case, most organizations are happy to provide you with details. The Web site www.clark.net/pub/pwalker/Fundraising_and_Giving/Foundations has listings of more than two dozen organizations that hold walkathons and similar charity events.

Here's one note of caution to walkathon participants: Make sure that the money you raise actually goes toward research and victim support rather than administrative purposes. It can be quite disheartening to find out that 80 percent of the money raised by an organization goes toward the salaries of the president and his administrative assistant. Before I sign up for a charitable event or before I contribute to other walkathon participants, I always ask an organization representative where the money goes.

Appendix

Walking Resources

• •

*I*f you want more information about any of the walking products, organizations, or publications mentioned in this book, check out this handy list of resources. Web surfers will be happy to know that I include Web sites for many of the resources.

ACE (American Council on Exercise)
5820 Oberlin Dr., Ste. 102
San Diego, CA 92121-3787
Phone: 800-825-3636
Web site: www.acefitness.org/

ACSM (American College of Sports Medicine)
P.O. Box 1440
Indianapolis, IN 46206-1440
Phone: 317-637-9200
Fax: 317-634-7817

Adidas
P.O. Box 4015
Beaverton, OR 97076-4015
Phone: 503-972-2300
Web site: www.adidas.com

AFAA (Aerobics and Fitness Association of America)
15250 Ventura Blvd., Ste. 200
Sherman Oaks, CA 91403
Phone: 800-225-2322

A.I. Stretch Rope
Maximum Performance International
51 W. 81st St.
New York, NY 10024
Phone: 212-799-7559

American Discovery Trail
P.O. Box 20155
Washington, DC 20041-2155
Phone: 800-663-2387 or 703-753-0149
Fax: 703-754-9008
E-mail: adtsociety@aol.com
Web site: www.discoverytrail.org

American Volkssport Association
1001 Pat Booker Rd., Suite 101
Universal City, TX 78148
Phone: 210-659-2112
Fax: 210-659-1212
E-mail: AVAHQ@aol.com
Web site: www.ava.org

Apex Fitness Equipment
#3-630 Esquimalt Rd.
Victoria, BC, Canada V9A 3L4
Phone: 250-381-4512 or 800-603-1655
Fax: 250-381-4582
E-mail: salesteam@apexfit.com
Web site: www.apexfit.com

Asics
ATTN: Consumer Relations
10540 Talbert Ave.
Fountain Valley, CA 92708
Phone: 800-678-9435
E-mail: consumer@asicstiger.com
Web site: www.asicstiger.com

Backroads
801 Cedar St.
Berkeley, CA 94710-1800
Phone: 800-GO-ACTIVE (800-462-2848)
Fax: 510-527-1444
Web site: www.backroads.com

Bioenergetics
200 Industrial Dr.
Birmingham, AL 35211
Phone: 800-433-2627

Blackburn
Bicycle Renaissance (dealer)
430 Columbus Ave.
New York, NY 10024
Phone: 212-724-2350

CamelBak Products, Inc.
1310 Redwood Way
Ste. 200
Petaluma, CA 94954
Phone: 800-767-8725 or 707-972-9700
Web site: www.camelbak.com

Champion (Jogbra)
5 New England Dr.
Essex, VT 05452
Phone: 888-301-5151
Web site: www.championforwomen.com

Collage Video
5390 Main St. NE
Minneapolis, MN 55421-1128
Phone: 800-433-6769
Web site: www.collagevideo.com

Cooking Light
2100 Lakeshore Dr.
Birmingham, AL 35209
Phone: 205-877-6000 or 800-336-0125
E-mail: cookinglight@spc.com
Web site: www.cookinglight.com

Cooper Institute for Aerobics Research
12330 Preston Rd.
Dallas, TX 75230
Phone: 800-635-7050
Web site: www.cooperinst.org

D.C. Walking Tours
2844 Wisconsin Ave., NW, Ste.310
Washington, DC 20007
Phone: 202-237-7534
Fax: 202-237-7468
E-mail: tourdc@dcwalkingtours.com
Web site: www.dcwalkingtours.com

Dupont (CoolMax)
Phone: 800-342-3774
E-mail: Dacron-Info.Janice-Baker@usa.dupont.com
Web site: www.dupont.com

Eagle Creek
3055 Enterprise Ct.
Vista, CA 92083
Phone: 800-874-9925
Web site: www.eaglecreek.com

Eastpak
900 Chelmsford St.
Lowell, MA 01851-8113
Phone: 978-454-4300

European Ramblers Association (ERA)
Generalsekretariat
Wilhelmshöher Allee 157-159
D-34121 Kassel
Germany

Exerstriders
P.O. Box 3313
Madison, WI 53704
Phone: 800-554-0989
Web site: www.exerstrider.com

E-Zone Networks
630 Airpark Rd., Ste. A
Napa, CA 94558
Phone: 707-259-1377
Fax: 707-259-1376
E-mail: sales@ezonenetworks.com
Web site: www.ezonenetworks.com

Family Circle
G+J Publishing USA
375 Lexington Ave.
New York, NY 10017
Web site: www.familycircle.com

Fitness Magazine
375 Lexington Ave.
New York, NY 10017-5514
Web site: www.fitnessmagazine.com

Fitness Partner Connection
Web site: www.primusweb.com/fitness partner/

FitnessLink
113 Circle Dr. S.
Lambertville, NJ 08530
Phone: 609-397-7664
Web site: www.fitnesslink.com

Flexaball
MegaFitness.com
P.O. Box 33536
Indialantic, FL 32903
Phone: 800-413-9942
Web site: www.megafitness.com

The Friendly Trails Travel Club
5457 Enberend Terrace
Columbia, MD 21045
Phone: 410-715-0912
Fax: 410-992-4665
Web site: www.harb.net/BAUERTRAVEL

Gym Source
40 E. 52nd St.
New York, NY 10022
Phone: 212-688-4222
Fax: 212-750-2886
Web site: www.gymsource.com

Health for Life
8033 Sunset Blvd., Ste. 483
Los Angeles, CA 90046
Phone: 800-874-5339 or 310-306-0777
Fax: 310-305-7672
E-mail: mail@healthforlife.com
Web site: www.healthforlife.com

Health World
Web site: www.healthy.net

IFE (Interactive Fitness Environment)
XYSTOS
1515 St. Jean-Baptiste St., Ste. 187
Quebec City, Quebec
Canada G2E 5E2
Phone: 877-4-XYSTOS
Web site: www.xystos.com

iVillage
Web site: www.iVillage.com

Jog-Bra
(*See* Champion)

Keiser Stretching Unit
Keiser Corp.
2470 S. Cherry Ave.
Fresno, CA 93706
Phone: 553-256-8000 or 800-888-7009
Fax: 559-256-8100
E-mail: sales@keiser.com
Web site: www.keiser.com

Landice, Inc.
111 Canfield Ave.
Randolph, NJ 07869-1114
Phone: 973-927-9010 or 800-LAN-DICE
Fax: 973-927-0630
Web site: www.landice.com

Lontex
P.O. Box 254
Perkasie, PA 18944
Phone: 800-343-8960
E-mail: sweatitout@prodigy.net
Web site: www.sweatitout.com

Men's Fitness
21100 Erwin St.
Woodland Hills, CA 91367
Phone: 818-884-6800
Web site: www.mensfitness.com

Men's Health
33 E. Minor St.
Emmaus, PA 18098
Phone: 610-967-8376
Web site: www.menshealth.com

The Method
The Balanced Body Center
232 Mercer St.
New York, NY 10012
Phone: 212-677-8416

The Mining Company
Web site: walking.miningco.com

CDNOW
Web site: www.cdnow.com

NASM (National Academy of Sports Medicine)
123 Hodencamp Dr., Ste. 204
Thousand Oaks, CA 91360
Phone: 800-656-2739
Fax: 805-449-1370

National Organization of Mall Walkers
P.O. Box 191
Hermann, MO 65041
Phone: 573-486-3945

National Safety Council
1121 Spring Lake Dr.
Itasca, IL 60143-3201
Phone: 630-285-1121
Fax: 630-285-1315
Web site: www.nsc.org

National Strength and Conditioning Association
1955 N. Union Blvd.
Colorado Springs, CO 80909
Phone: 719-632-6722
Fax: 719-632-6367
E-mail: nsca@nsca-lift.org

Net Pulse Communications, Inc.
215 Second St., 3rd Fl.
San Francisco, CA 94105
Phone: 415-357-1999
Fax: 415-357-1998
E-mail: info@netpulse.net
Web site: www.netpulse.net

New Balance Athletic Shoe
61 N. Beacon St.
Boston, MA 02134
Phone: 617-783-4000 or 800-NBF-STOR
Fax: 617-787-9355 or 617-783-5152
Web site: www.newbalance.com

New York Road Runners Club
9 E. 89th St.
New York, NY 10128
Phone: 212-423-2238
Web site: www.nyrrc.org

Nike
One Bowerman Dr.
Beaverton, OR 97005
Phone: 800-806-6453
Web site: www.nike.com

Paragon
867 Broadway
New York, NY 10003
Phone: 212-255-8036 or 800-961-3030
Web site: www.paragonsports.com

Partnership for a Walkable America
(*See* National Safety Council)

Patagonia
8550 White Fir St.
P.O. Box 32050
Reno, NV 89523
Phone: 800-638-6464
Web site: www.patagonia.com

Physical Genius, Inc.
1105 Taylorsville Rd.
Washington Crossing, PA 18977
Phone: 215-369-9830
Fax: 215-369-9832
Web site: www.physicalgenius.com

Physical Mind Institute
1807 Second St. Ste. 15
Santa Fe, NM 87505
Phone: 505-988-1990
Fax: 505-988-2837
Web site: www.the-method.com

Physioballs
Resist-A-Ball
6435 Castleway W. Dr.
Ste. 130
Indianapolis, IN 46250
Phone: 317-576-6571
Fax: 317-576-6575

Pilates Studio, The
2121 Broadway, Ste. 201
New York, NY 10023
Phone: 800-474-5283
Fax: 212-769-2368

Polar Electro, Inc.
(Polar Heart Monitor)
370 Crossways Park Dr.
Woodbury, NY 11797-2050
Phone: 516-364-0400 or 800-227-1314
Fax: 516-364-5454
Web site: www.polar.usa.com

Precor, Inc.
Commercial Products Division
20001 N. Creek Pky.
P.O. Box 3004
Bothell, WA 98041-3004
Phone: 425-486-9292 or 800-786-8404
Fax: 425-486-3856
Web site: www.precor.com

President's Council on Physical Fitness & Sports
200 Independence Ave. S.W., Room 738H
Washington, DC 20201
Phone: 202-690-9000
Fax: 202-690-5211

Prevention Magazine
33 E. Minor St.
Emmaus, PA 18098
Phone: 610-967-5171
Web site: www.prevention.com

Prostretch/Prism
6952 Fairgrounds Pky.
San Antonio, TX 78238
Phone: 210-520-8051 or 800-535-6329
Fax: 210-520-8039
Web site: www.prostretch.com

Quinton Fitness Equipment
Quinton Instruments Co.
3303 Monte Villa Pky.
Bothell, WA 98021
Phone: 425-402-2000 or 800-426-0337, ext. 2440
Fax: 425-402-2009
Web site: www.quinton.com

RaceReady Clothing catalog
Phone: 800-537-6868
Web site: www.raceready.com

Racewalk.com
Web site: www.racewalk.com

Redbook
224 W. 57th St.
New York, NY 10019
Phone: 212-649-3450
Web site: http://redbook.women.com/rb/

Reebok Int'l Ltd.
1000 Technology Center Dr.
Stoughton, MA 02072-4705
Phone: 800-REE-BOK1
Fax: 717-687-6987
Web site: www.reebok.com

Road Runner Sports
5549 Copley Dr.
San Diego, CA 92111
Phone: 800-636-3560
Fax: 800-453-5443
Web site: www.roadrunnersports.com

Rockport
Div. Reebok
220 Donald Lynch Blvd.
Marlborough, MA 01752
Phone: 508-485-2090 or 800-762-5767
Fax: 508-480-0012
Web site: www.rockport.com

Ryka
555 S. Henderson Rd.
King of Prussia, PA 19406-3514
Phone: 800-255-RYKA
Fax: 610-768-0753
Web site: www.ryka.com

Saucony
13 Centennial Dr.
Peabody, MA 01961
Phone: 978-532-9000 or 800-365-4933
Web site: www.saucony.com

Sawyer Products
(Makers of insect repellents, sunblocks, and treatments
for bites and stings)
Phone: 800-940-4464
Web site: www.sawyerproducts.com

Shape Magazine
21100 Irwin St.
Woodland Hills, CA 91367
Phone: 818-884-6800
Fax: 818-704-7620
Web site: www.shapeonline.com

SmartWool
40250 County Rd. 129
Steamboat Springs, CO 80487
Phone: 970-879-2913 or 800-550-9665
Fax: 970-879-0937
Web site: www.smartwool.com

Specialty Travel Index ONLINE
305 San Anselmo Ave., Suite 313
San Anselmo, CA 94960
Phone: 415-455-1643 or 888-624-4030
Fax: 415-459-4974
E-mail: spectrav@ix.netcom.com
Web site: www.specialtytravel.com

Spenco Medical Corp.
6301 Imperial Dr.
Waco, TX 76712
Phone: 254-772-6000 or 800-877-3626
Web site: www.spenco.com

Star Trac by Unisen, Inc.
14410 Myford Rd.
Irvine, CA 92606
Phone: 714-669-1660 or 800-228-6635

Step Co.
1395 S. Marietta Pkwy., Bldg. 200
Marietta, GA 30067
Phone: 800-SAY-STEP
Fax: 770-424-1590

Stretching, Inc.
P.O. Box 767
Palmer Lake, CO 80133-0767
Phone: 719-481-3928 or 800-333-1307
Fax: 719-781-9058
E-mail: office@stretching.com
Web site: www.stretching.com

Teva Sport Sandals
P.O. Box 968
Flagstaff, AZ 86002
Phone: 800-367-8382
Fax: 520-779-6004
Web site: www.tevasandals.com

Thor-Lo Inc.
P.O. Box 5399
Statesville, NC 28687-5399
Phone: 800-457-2256
Fax: 704-838-6323
Web site: www.thorlo.com

The Timex Corporation
P.O. Box 310
Middlebury, CT 06762
Phone: 203-573-5000
Web site: www.timex.com

Title Nine Sports
5743 Landragan St.
Emeryville, CA 94608
Phone: 800-609-0092
Fax: 510-655-9191
E-mail: thefolks@title9sports.com
Web site: www.title9sports.com

TOPS (Take Off Pounds Sensibly), Inc.
4575 S. Fifth St.
P.O. Box 07360
Milwaukee, WI 53207-0360
Phone: 414-482-4620 or 800-932-8677
Web site: www.tops.org

Trotter (CYBEX)
10 Trotter Dr.
Medway, MA 02053
Phone: 508-533-4300 or 888-GOC-YBEX
Web site: www.cybexintl.com

True Fitness
865 Hoff Rd.
O'Fallon, MO 63366
Phone: 800-426-6570
Fax: 314-272-7148
Web site: www.truefitness.com

Tune Belt, Inc.
11400 Grooms Rd.
Cincinnati, OH 45242
Phone: 800-860-1175 or 513-247-4400
Fax: 513-247-4410

U.S. Department of Transportation
Bureau of Transportation Services
General information: 202-366-3282
Web site: www.dot.gov

U.S. Fish and Wildlife Service
Web site: www.fws.gov

The Walking Connection
www.walkingconnection.com/Walk_Members_Home_Page.html

Walking Magazine
Subscription Office
P.O. Box 5073
Harlan, IA 51593
Phone: 800-829-5585
Web site: www.walkingmag.com

Wigwam
3402 Crocker Ave.
Sheboygan, WI 53081
Phone: 920-457-5551 or 800-558-7760
Fax: 920-457-0311
Web site: www.wigwam.com

Women.com Walking Clubs
Web site: www.women.com/clubs/walking.html

YMCA of the USA
101 N. Wacker Dr.
Chicago, IL 60606
Phone: 312-977-0031
Fax: 312-977-9063
Web site: www.ymca.net

Index

• *E* •

• G •

• *H* •

• Q •

• R •

• *S* •

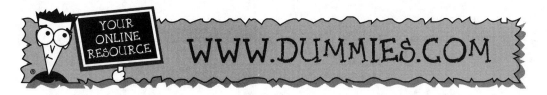

YOUR ONLINE RESOURCE

WWW.DUMMIES.COM

Discover Dummies Online!

The Dummies Web Site is your fun and friendly online resource for the latest information about ...*For Dummies*® books and your favorite topics. The Web site is the place to communicate with us, exchange ideas with other ...*For Dummies* readers, chat with authors, and have fun!

Ten Fun and Useful Things You Can Do at www.dummies.com

1. Win free ...*For Dummies* books and more!
2. Register your book and be entered in a prize drawing.
3. Meet your favorite authors through the IDG Books Author Chat Series.
4. Exchange helpful information with other ...*For Dummies* readers.
5. Discover other great ...*For Dummies* books you must have!
6. Purchase Dummieswear™ exclusively from our Web site.
7. Buy ...*For Dummies* books online.
8. Talk to us. Make comments, ask questions, get answers!
9. Download free software.
10. Find additional useful resources from authors.

Link directly to these ten fun and useful things at **http://www.dummies.com/10useful**

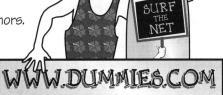

WWW.DUMMIES.COM

For other technology titles from IDG Books Worldwide, go to **www.idgbooks.com**

Not on the Web yet? It's easy to get started with *Dummies 101*®: *The Internet For Windows*® *98* or *The Internet For Dummies*®, 6th Edition, at local retailers everywhere.

IDG BOOKS WORLDWIDE

Find other ...*For Dummies* books on these topics:
Business • Career • Databases • Food & Beverage • Games • Gardening • Graphics • Hardware
Health & Fitness • Internet and the World Wide Web • Networking • Office Suites
Operating Systems • Personal Finance • Pets • Programming • Recreation • Sports
Spreadsheets • Teacher Resources • Test Prep • Word Processing

IDG BOOKS WORLDWIDE
BOOK REGISTRATION

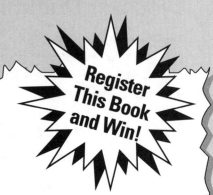

Register This Book and Win!

We want to hear from you!

Visit **http://my2cents.dummies.com** to register this book and tell us how you liked it!

- ✔ Get entered in our monthly prize giveaway.

- ✔ Give us feedback about this book — tell us what you like best, what you like least, or maybe what you'd like to ask the author and us to change!

- ✔ Let us know any other *...For Dummies*® topics that interest you.

Your feedback helps us determine what books to publish, tells us what coverage to add as we revise our books, and lets us know whether we're meeting your needs as a *...For Dummies* reader. You're our most valuable resource, and what you have to say is important to us!

Not on the Web yet? It's easy to get started with *Dummies 101*®: *The Internet For Windows*® *98* or *The Internet For Dummies*®, 6th Edition, at local retailers everywhere.

Or let us know what you think by sending us a letter at the following address:

...For Dummies Book Registration
Dummies Press
7260 Shadeland Station, Suite 100
Indianapolis, IN 46256-3917
Fax 317-596-5498

BESTSELLING BOOK SERIES